Diabetic Kidney Disease

Takashi Wada • Kengo Furuichi
Naoki Kashihara
Editors

Diabetic Kidney Disease

Springer

Editors
Takashi Wada
Department of Nephrology and Laboratory
Kanazawa University
Kanazawa, Ishikawa
Japan

Kengo Furuichi
Department of Nephrology
Kanazawa Medical University
Kanazawa, Ishikawa
Japan

Naoki Kashihara
Department of Nephrology and Hypertension
Kawasaki Medical School
Kurashiki, Okayama
Japan

ISBN 978-981-15-9303-1 ISBN 978-981-15-9301-7 (eBook)
https://doi.org/10.1007/978-981-15-9301-7

This Springer imprint is published by the registered company Springer Nature Singapore Pte Ltd.
The registered company address is: 152 Beach Road, #21-01/04 Gateway East, Singapore 189721, Singapore

Preface

Diabetic kidney disease is the leading cause of end-stage kidney disease requiring renal replacement therapy. Nowadays, the circumstances in aging society affect and alter the clinico-pathological phenotypes and kidney prognosis in diabetic patients. With these trends, the terms of diabetic kidney disease may be used for clinical approach for diabetes-related kidney disease, in which further discussion would be required for pathophysiology, therapy, and prognosis.

The purpose of this book is to provide the latest information on clinico-pathological features of diabetic kidney disease, especially based on results from a cohort of biopsy-proven diabetic nephropathy patients with long-term medical observation and long-term registry for diabetic kidney disease and recent progress in pathophysiology. Biopsy-proven diabetic nephropathy cohort increases the value of clinical and experimental settings. Therefore, these will clearly provide the readers with clinico-pathological axis in clinical and experimental settings, including differential pathological/clinical diagnoses of chronic kidney disease in diabetic patients (e.g., the presence of "classical" diabetic nephropathy and/or nephrosclerosis and/or other primary kidney diseases). Therefore, the description of this book is very informative for all physicians and researchers all over the world in this field.

We gratefully thank all contributors for preparing their manuscripts and chapters for a better understanding of the current status of diabetic kidney disease. We are further thankful to Springer Nature, especially Vignesh Iyyadurai Suresh and Sachiko Hayakawa for their patience and invaluable advice.

Kanazawa, Japan — Takashi Wada
Kanazawa, Japan — Kengo Furuichi
Kurashiki, Japan — Naoki Kashihara

Contents

Part II Pathological Aspects

Part I
Clinical Aspects

Chapter 1
Clinical Epidemiology

Tadashi Toyama

DKD is a disease concept that has received much attention in recent years. The definition of DKD is not yet well established and may vary from studies. On the other hand, the importance of DKD as a risk factor, its high incidence, or a specific condition such as normoalbuminuric DKD is getting a lot of attention. This chapter outlines the definition of DKD, its role as a risk factor, the international incidence of the disease, and characteristics of normoalbuminuric DKD.

1.1 Definition of DKD

Diabetic nephropathy is clinically diagnosed when the major features of diabetic nephropathy, albuminuria (>300 mg/24 h or 200 μg/min), and diabetic retinopathy are found and other kidney diseases are excluded [1]. Studies have revealed that not only albuminuria but also reduced GFR is a risk factor for ESKD and cardiovascular diseases (CVD) [2, 3]. Furthermore, in recent years, diabetic patients with reduced GFR and normoalbuminuria have been increasing [4]. Due to such clinical evidence and changes in disease structure, the concept of disease called DKD, which is a CKD with diabetes, has become widespread. There is no widely accepted definition of DKD, but American Diabetes Association (ADA) said "DKD is usually a clinical diagnosis made based on the presence of albuminuria and/or reduced eGFR in the absence of sign or symptoms of other primary causes of kidney damage" [5].

DKD is a major microvascular complication of diabetes. Increasing number of ESKD requiring dialysis or kidney transplantation is a worldwide burden, and DKD is a major cause of ESKD in many high-income or upper-middle-income countries.

T. Toyama (✉)
Division of Nephrology, Kanazawa University Hospital, Kanazawa, Japan
e-mail: t-toyama@staff.kanazawa-u.ac.jp

T. Wada et al. (eds.), *Diabetic Kidney Disease*,
https://doi.org/10.1007/978-981-15-9301-7_1

1.2 Prevalence of Diabetes

The International Diabetes Federation reported that the prevalence of diabetes in global estimates was 9.3% (Fig. 1.1), and 463.0 million adults aged 20–79 years are suffering from diabetes [6]. The total number of diabetes has been increasing worldwide [7]. Considering the global situation of diabetes, concern about the future burden of DKD is increasing.

1.3 Incidence of DKD

The United Kingdom Prospective Diabetes Study (UKPDS 64) followed 5097 patients with type 2 diabetes and revealed annual incidence of DKD by its stage [8] (Fig. 1.2). The incidence rates of normoalbuminuria to microalbuminuria, microalbuminuria to macroalbuminuria, and macroalbuminuria to ESKD were 2.0%, 2.8%, and 2.3%, respectively. It is noteworthy that the all-cause mortality rate is equal to or greater than the progression rate of nephropathy. As reported in other studies, the most common cause of death is cardiovascular disease (CVD), and

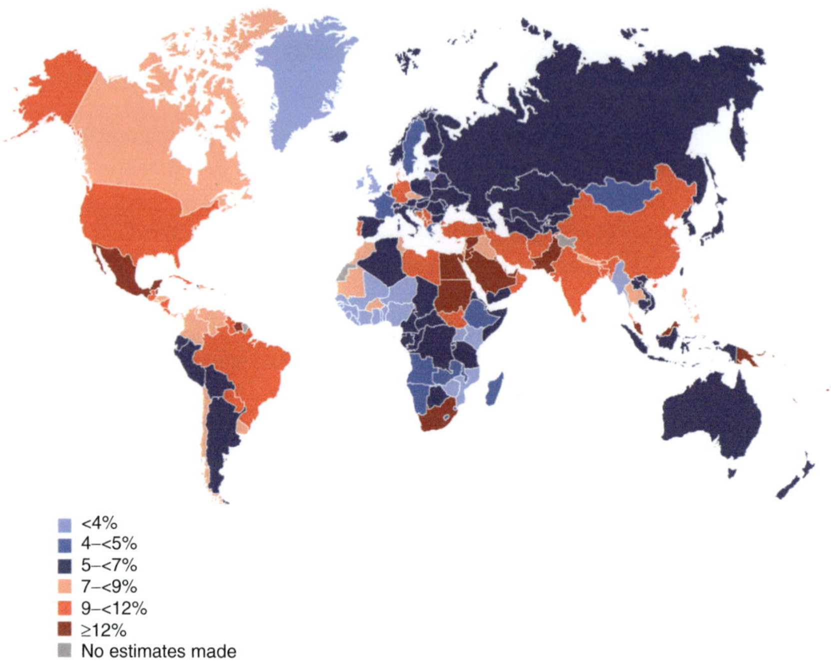

Fig. 1.1 Estimated age-adjusted prevalence of diabetes in adults (20–79 years), 2019 [7]

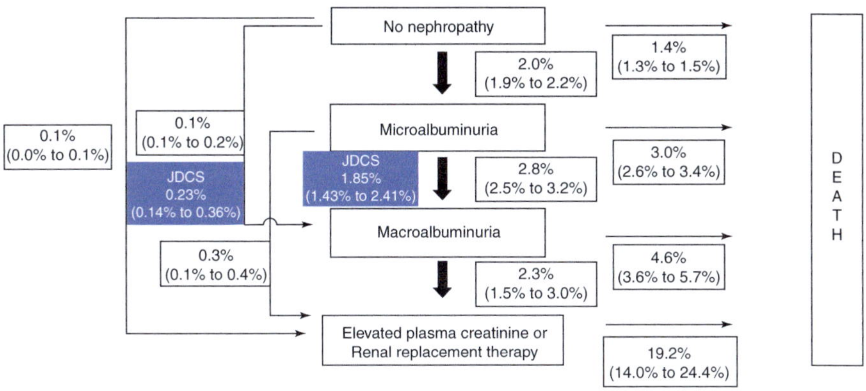

Fig. 1.2 Annual transition rates through the stages of nephropathy and to death from any cause [8, 11]. Figure of UKPDS was partially modified with information of JDCS

albuminuria is considered one of the major risk factors for CVD [2, 9]. In a cohort study of Taiwan, early DKD (diabetes in CKD stage 1–3) was related to a 16-year loss in life expectancy compared to diabetes without CKD [10].

The Japan Diabetes Complications Study (JDCS), a study of Japanese patients with type 2 diabetes with a mean diabetes duration of 10.7 years, reported that 1.85% annual changes from low-microalbuminuria (3.4–17.0 mg/mmol) to macroalbuminuria and 0.23% annual changes from normoalbuminuria to macroalbuminuria [11], which is almost the same incidence in UKPDS (Fig. 1.2).

1.4 Incidence of ESRD in DKD Patients

In Japan, where the prevalence of maintenance dialysis patients is secondarily high followed by Taiwan [12], diabetes has been the most common primary disease for ESKD in patients requiring dialysis since 1998. Although the rate of diabetes causing ESKD reached a plateau, 42.3% of those who start dialysis had diabetes as the primary disease [13] (Fig. 1.3).

Diabetes is the most common primary cause of ESKD in the United States as well. This rate has not changed significantly over the past 20 years but has been increasing progressively, and in 2017 it was 48.1% (Fig. 1.4).

In international comparisons, Malaysia, Singapore, and Jalisco (Mexico) were the countries with the highest rates of diabetes as a cause of ESRD in 2016 at approximately 66% [12]. Following them, in many high-income countries including Japan, the United States, South Korea, Israel, Hong Kong, and New Zealand, approximately 50% of the causes of ESRD are diabetes [12].

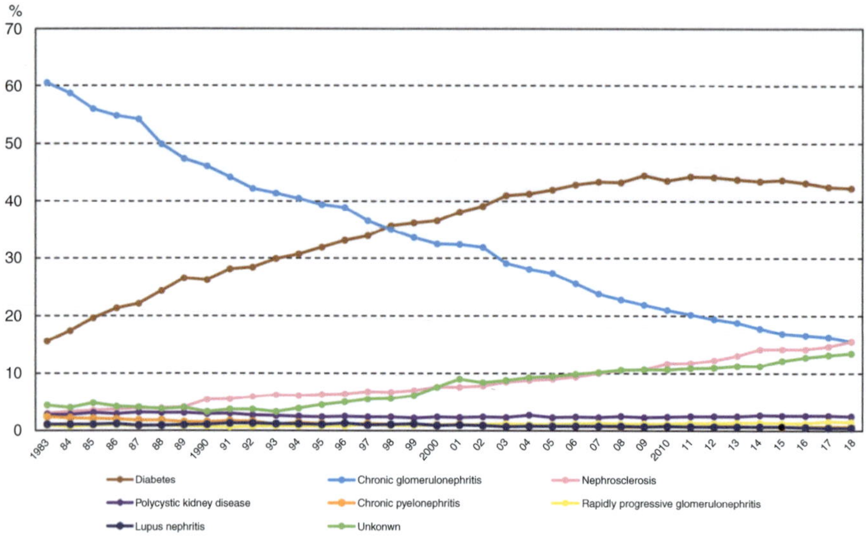

Fig. 1.3 Changes in proportion of primary cause of end-stage kidney disease in patients initiating dialysis in Japan (the data reported here have been provided by the Japanese Society for Dialysis Therapy (JSDT). The interpretation and reporting of these data are the responsibility of the authors and in no way should be seen as an official policy or interpretation of the JSDT) [13]

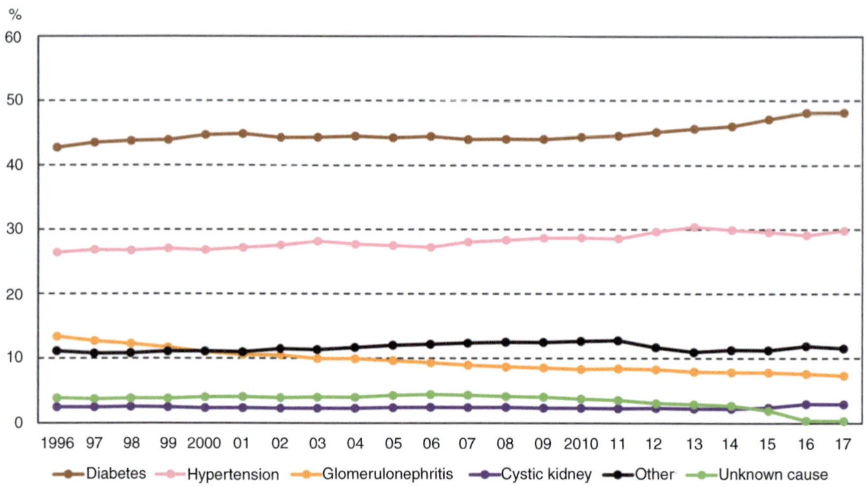

Fig. 1.4 Changes in proportion of primary cause of end-stage kidney disease in patients initiating dialysis in the United States created from data provided in USRDS [12]

1.5 Prevalence of DKD

Table 1.1 shows the prevalence of albuminuria and DKD in representative type 2 diabetes cohorts. Prevalence of albuminuria is listed as the main manifestation of kidney damage in diabetes. The UKPDS study reported that, in patients with type 2 diabetes 10 years after diagnosis, the prevalence of microalbuminuria, macroalbuminuria, and elevated plasma creatinine or renal replacement therapy were 24.9%, 5.3%, and 0.8%, respectively [8]. In the analysis of National Health and Nutrition Examination Survey (NHANES), the cohort study of US population, the prevalence of DKD (albuminuria and/or reduced eGFR) in NHANES 2009–2014 adults with diabetes was 25% [14].

Asians were reported to have a high incidence of albuminuria. In the MacroAlbuminuria Prevalence (MAP) study, including Chinese and Filipino, the mean duration of type 2 diabetes was 6.9 years, the prevalence rate of microalbuminuria was 39.8%, and the macroalbuminuria was 18.8% [15]. In Developing Education on Microalbuminuria for Awareness of reNal and cardiovascular risk in Diabetes (DEMAND), microalbuminuria and DKD showed prevalence of 38.8% and 57.3%, respectively [16]. In this study, Caucasians, who accounted for 39% of the participants, had a prevalence of microalbuminuria of 33%, lower than those of other ethnicities [16]. In the Japan Diabetes Clinical Data Management study (JDDM), the prevalence of DKD in Japanese population was 43.8% [17].

In studies of type 1 diabetes, a cohort study in the Steno Memorial Hospital reported that cumulative prevalence of diabetic nephropathy was 45% after 40 years of diabetes [18]. The Diabetes Control and Complications Trial/Epidemiology of Diabetes Interventions and Complications (DCCT/EDIC) reported that the cumulative incidence of microalbuminuria in 30 years was 25% or 38% for intensive and conventional diabetes therapy, respectively [19]. The cumulative proportion of diabetic nephropathy in patients with type 1 diabetes has showed decreasing trend from 1961 to 1985 [20]. It might be because many patients were treated according to the evidence of tight glycemic control [21].

To date, many evidence-based treatments for DKD have been clarified and applied in clinical practice. Poor glucose control has been noted as a major risk factor for DKD [22, 23], and a number of glucose-lowering agents have been launched during the several decades. Angiotensin-converting enzyme (ACE) inhibitors and angiotensin II receptor blockers (ARBs), reported to suppress the onset and progression of DKD [24–26], are widely used. In addition, studies showed the effectiveness of sodium-glucose cotransporter-2 (SGLT2) inhibitors on DKD, and it is expected to suppress the DKD onset [27–29] and progression [30]. However, an obvious reduction in the prevalence of DKD was not observed. In the real world, the effect of treatments in the interventional trials might be attenuated and nearly 50% of diabetic patients achieved HbA1c < 7.0% [31]. In order to reduce the residual risk, a detailed pathophysiology and a treatment strategy based on this are required.

Table 1.1 Prevalence of albuminuria and DKD in representative type 2 diabetic cohorts

Study	Race	Analysis year	Mean duration of diabetes (years)	Microalbuminuria (%)	Macroalbuminuria (%)	DKD (albuminuria and/or reduced GFR)
UKPDS [8]	White 82% Others 18%	2002	10	24.9	5.3	NA
MAP [15] (*n* = 5549)	Chinese 59% Malay 14% Filipino 21% Others 6%	2005	6.9	39.8	18.8	NA
DEMAND [16] (*n* = 24,151)	Caucasian 39% Asian 38% Hispanic 5%	2006	7.6	38.8	9.8	57.3%[a]
JDDM [17] (*n* = 8897)	Japanese 100%	2007	12	31.6	10.5[a]	43.8%[a]
NHANES [14] (*n* = 2279)	White 60% Black 15% Mexican American 10%	2009–2014	5.0[b]	16[c]	4.6	25%

[a]Calculated from the data provided in the article
[b]Median duration of diabetes
[c]Defined as albumin-to-creatinine ratio $\geq$ 30 mg/g
Abbreviations: *DKD* diabetic kidney disease, *NA* not available

1.6 DKD Without Albuminuria

Albuminuria and reduced GFR are both definition of DKD and risk factors for ESKD, CVD, and all-cause mortality [2, 3, 9]. In recent years, the prevalance of albuminuria and reduced GFR has changed. DKD population analysis in NHANES since 1988 showed a decrease in the proportion of albuminuria and an increase in the proportion of reduced GFR [4]. The United States Renal Data System (USRDS) reported that in NHANES participants nearly a quarter of diabetic patients with CKD had reduced eGFR (<60 mL/min/1.73 m^2) without albuminuria (Fig. 1.5) [12].

Cohort studies of diabetic patients revealed that reduced GFR without albuminuria related increased risks of ESRD or all-cause mortality [2, 3, 9]. It should be noted when accompanied by albuminuria, even a moderate decline in eGFR (30–59 mL/min/1.73 m^2) significantly increases the risk of kidney events and all-cause mortality (Table 1.2). Reduced GFR without albuminuria showed a mild trend toward a risk of all-cause mortality (Table 1.2, Fig. 1.6).

The importance of albuminuria was confirmed in biopsy-proven DKD. In a study of 82 cases of biopsy-proven DKD, nonproteinuric DKD had less-frequent typical pathological lesions and a lower risk of CKD progression and mortality compared to proteinuric DKD [32] (Fig. 1.7).

Other cohort studies have reported that normoalbuminuria is associated with atherosclerotic lesions rather than diabetes-related renal lesions. In the JDDM, 262 (11.4%) of 2298 Japanese type 2 diabetic patients with normoalbuminuria had reduced renal function (eGFR <60 mL/min/1.72 m^2), and 63.4% of them did not

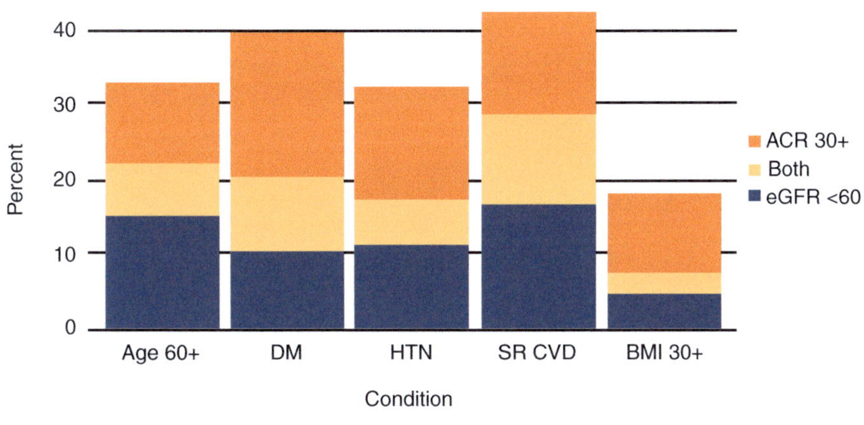

Fig. 1.5 Distribution of markers of CKD in NHANES participants with diabetes, hypertension, self-reported cardiovascular disease, and obesity, 2011–2014 [12]. Data Source: National Health and Nutrition Examination Survey (NHANES), 2011–2014 participants age 20 and older. Single-sample estimates of eGFR and ACR; eGFR calculated using the CKD-EPI equation. Abbreviations: *ACR* urine albumin/creatinine ratio, *BMI* body mass index, *CKD* chronic kidney disease, *SR CVD* self-reported cardiovascular disease, *eGFR* estimated glomerular filtration rate, *HTN* hypertension

Table 1.2 Hazard ratios based on CKD stages for each outcome [2]

UACR	eGFR (mL/min/1.73 m^2)						*p* for trend (eGFR)
	>90	60–89	45–59	30–44	15–29	<15	
Renal events (RRT or halving reduced eGFR)							
Normoalbuminuria	1.00 (Reference)	1.00 (Reference)	0.69 (0.24–1.98)	1.83 (0.53–6.31)	11.59 (1.43–93.78)	NA	0.85
Microalbuminuria	3.31 (2.07–5.28)	3.04 (1.98–4.68)	3.36 (1.63–6.93)	3.10 (1.41–6.83)	3.60 (0.42–31.28)	NA	0.60
Macroalbuminuria	11.14 (5.87–21.17)	15.64 (10.30–23.74)	33.37 (20.58–50.91)	41.36 (25.09–68.16)	71.58 (40.41–126.80)	NA	<0.01
p for trend (albuminuria)	<0.01	<0.01	<0.01	<0.01	0.06	NA	
Cardiovascular events							
Normoalbuminuria	1.00 (Reference)	1.00 (Reference)	1.05 (0.73–1.49)	1.30 (0.74–2.28)	0.42 (0.06–3.06)	NA	0.46
Microalbuminuria	1.01 (0.69–1.49)	1.48 (1.15–1.90)	1.33 (0.89–2.00)	1.85 (1.20–2.85)	0.47 (0.11–1.97)	NA	0.04
Macroalbuminuria	1.28 (0.56–2.94)	2.10 (1.46–3.02)	1.85 (1.23–2.78)	2.37 (1.55–3.63)	2.09 (1.26–3.45)	12.76 (0.95–171.19)	0.20
p for trend (albuminuria)	0.81	<0.01	0.09	0.45	0.17	NA	
All-cause mortality							
Normoalbuminuria	1.00 (Reference)	1.00 (Reference)	1.67 (1.02–2.74)	1.22 (0.43–3.46)	8.19 (2.65–25.34)	NA	<0.01
Microalbuminuria	1.51 (0.78–2.95)	1.44 (0.92–2.24)	1.22 (0.63–2.35)	0.84 (0.31–2.26)	8.36 (2.81–24.90)	NA	0.04
Macroalbuminuria	4.37 (1.70–11.24)	1.92 (0.97–3.79)	4.84 (2.72–8.62)	4.09 (2.00–8.34)	6.16 (2.80–13.56)	70.57 (3.65–1363.68)	0.06
p for trend (albuminuria)	0.01	0.01	0.01	0.02	0.80	NA	

The estimates are adjusted for age, gender, HbA1c, and systolic blood pressure

Abbreviations: *UACR* urine albumin-to-creatinine ratio, *eGFR* estimated glomerular filtration rate, *RRT* renal replacement therapy, *NA* not available

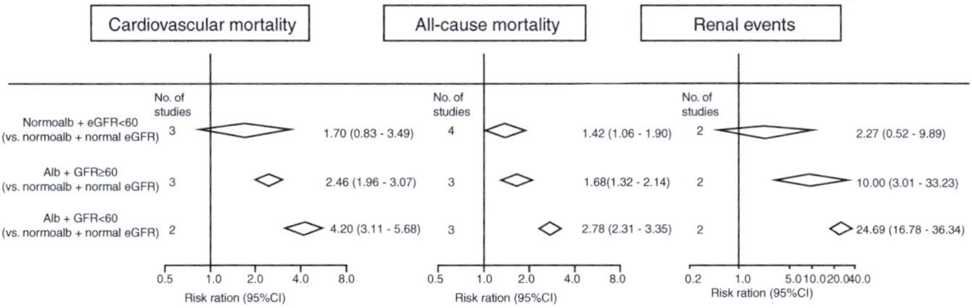

Fig. 1.6 Risk ratio for the association of low eGFR with the risk of each outcome according to the presence of albuminuria, compared with normal eGFR and normoalbuminuria. Albuminuria was defined as any level of albuminuria or pooled estimate of microalbuminuria and macroalbuminuria. Abbreviations: *normoalb* normoalbuminuria, *alb* albuminuria [3]

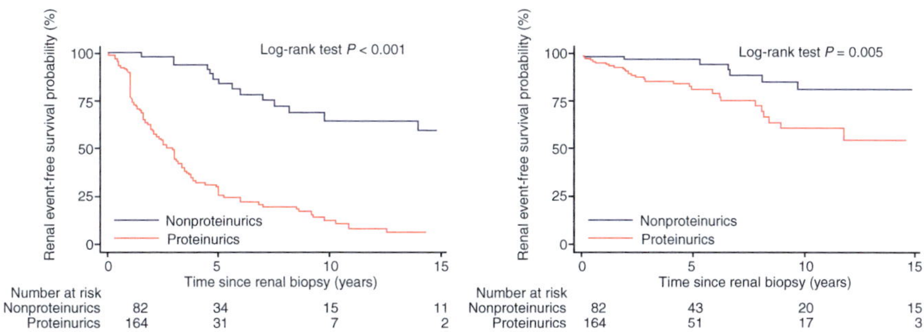

Fig. 1.7 Renal event-free survival for the 164 patients of propensity-matched DKD cohort. Left: CKD progression-free survival. Right: death event-free survival [32]

have retinopathy nor neuropathy [33]. In this patient group, arteriosclerotic rather than diabetic lesion may be the cause of kidney injury. In a study of renal biopsy in 15 Japanese patients with diabetes who had normoalbuminuria and reduced eGFR, nine cases showed disproportionately advanced tubulointerstitial lesions, vascular lesions, and global glomerulosclerosis with minor diabetic glomerular lesion [34] (Fig. 1.8), which is category III of the patterns proposed by Fioretto [35].

An autopsy study reported that of 168 people clinically diagnosed diabetes, 106 (63%) of autopsy tissue specimen showed lesions consistent with diabetic nephropathy [36]. Interestingly, 20 of 106 patients with histologically proven diabetic nephropathy did not show albuminuria in their lifetime [36]. While the clinical diagnosis of DKD is important, the clinical implications of the pathological findings of DKD need to be more clarified in order to provide appropriate prevention and treatment options. Regarding this, the pathological definition has been announced from Japan [37], and the relation with the prognosis has been studied [38, 39]. For details, see Chaps. 9–11.

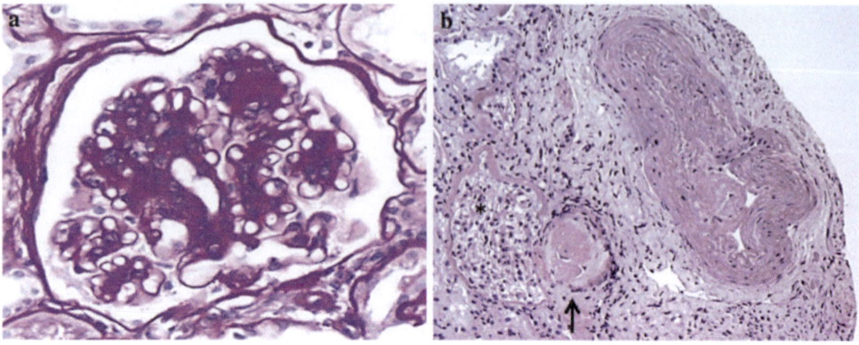

Fig. 1.8 Representative microscopic findings in type 2 diabetic patients with normoalbuminuria (normal proteinuria) and low eGFR (<60 mL/min/1.73 m^2). (**a**) Severe diffuse lesions in a patient classified as typical lesions of diabetic nephropathy (category II) (periodic acid-Schiff (PAS) stain ×200). (**b**) Mild diffuse lesions (asterisk) associated with global glomerular sclerosis (arrow) and disproportionately advanced arteriosclerosis, which denotes the presence of diabetic kidney lesions as well as nephrosclerosis, in a patient classified as atypical patterns (category III) (PAS stain ×100) [34]

1.7 Conclusion

Epidemiology of DKD is outlined in this chapter. The incidence and prevalence of DKD varies according to the definition of DKD and requires careful interpretation. Detailed observation of the pathophysiology of kidney disease associated with diabetes will provide evidence that can be used for treatment.

References

1. Skorecki K, Chertow GM, Marsden PA, Taal MW, Yu ASL. Brenner and Rector's the kidney. Philadelphia, PA: Elsevier; 2016.
2. Wada T, Haneda M, Furuichi K, Babazono T, Yokoyama H, Iseki K, et al. Clinical impact of albuminuria and glomerular filtration rate on renal and cardiovascular events, and all-cause mortality in Japanese patients with type 2 diabetes. Clin Exp Nephrol. 2014;18(4):613–20.
3. Toyama T, Furuichi K, Ninomiya T, Shimizu M, Hara A, Iwata Y, et al. The impacts of albuminuria and low eGFR on the risk of cardiovascular death, all-cause mortality, and renal events in diabetic patients: meta-analysis. PLoS One. 2013;8(8):e71810.
4. Afkarian M, Zelnick LR, Hall YN, Heagerty PJ, Tuttle K, Weiss NS, et al. Clinical manifestations of kidney disease among US adults with diabetes, 1988–2014. JAMA. 2016;316(6):602–10.
5. American Diabetes Association. 10. Microvascular complications and foot care: standards of medical care in diabetes-2018. Diabetes Care. 2018;41(Suppl 1):S105–S18.
6. IDF Diabetes Atlas, 8th edn. Brussels: International Diabetes Federation; 2017.
7. IDF Diabetes Atlas, 9th edn. Brussels: International Diabetes Federation; 2019.
8. Adler AI, Stevens RJ, Manley SE, Bilous RW, Cull CA, Holman RR, et al. Development and progression of nephropathy in type 2 diabetes: the United Kingdom Prospective Diabetes Study (UKPDS 64). Kidney Int. 2003;63(1):225–32.

9. Ninomiya T, Perkovic V, de Galan BE, Zoungas S, Pillai A, Jardine M, et al. Albuminuria and kidney function independently predict cardiovascular and renal outcomes in diabetes. J Am Soc Nephrol. 2009;20(8):1813–21.
10. Wen CP, Chang CH, Tsai MK, Lee JH, Lu PJ, Tsai SP, et al. Diabetes with early kidney involvement may shorten life expectancy by 16 years. Kidney Int. 2017;92(2):388–96.
11. Katayama S, Moriya T, Tanaka S, Tanaka S, Yajima Y, Sone H, et al. Low transition rate from normo- and low microalbuminuria to proteinuria in Japanese type 2 diabetic individuals: the Japan Diabetes Complications Study (JDCS). Diabetologia. 2011;54(5):1025–31.
12. United States Renal Data System. 2019 USRDS annual data report: epidemiology of kidney disease in the United States. Bethesda, MD: National Institutes of Health, National Institute of Diabetes and Digestive and Kidney Diseases; 2019.
13. Nitta K. 2018 Annual dialysis data report, JSDT renal data registry. Nihon Toseki Igakkai Zasshi. 2019;52(12):679–754.
14. Zelnick LR, Weiss NS, Kestenbaum BR, Robinson-Cohen C, Heagerty PJ, Tuttle K, et al. Diabetes and CKD in the United States population, 2009–2014. Clin J Am Soc Nephrol. 2017;12(12):1984–90.
15. Wu AY, Kong NC, de Leon FA, Pan CY, Tai TY, Yeung VT, et al. An alarmingly high prevalence of diabetic nephropathy in Asian type 2 diabetic patients: the MicroAlbuminuria Prevalence (MAP) Study. Diabetologia. 2005;48(1):17–26.
16. Parving HH, Lewis JB, Ravid M, Remuzzi G, Hunsicker LG, DEMAND Investigators. Prevalence and risk factors for microalbuminuria in a referred cohort of type II diabetic patients: a global perspective. Kidney Int. 2006;69(11):2057–63.
17. Yokoyama H, Kawai K, Kobayashi M, Japan Diabetes Clinical Data Management Study Group. Microalbuminuria is common in Japanese type 2 diabetic patients: a nationwide survey from the Japan Diabetes Clinical Data Management Study Group (JDDM 10). Diabetes Care. 2007;30(4):989–92.
18. Andersen AR, Christiansen JS, Andersen JK, Kreiner S, Deckert T. Diabetic nephropathy in type 1 (insulin-dependent) diabetes: an epidemiological study. Diabetologia. 1983;25(6):496–501.
19. de Boer IH, DCCT/EDIC Research Group. Kidney disease and related findings in the diabetes control and complications trial/epidemiology of diabetes interventions and complications study. Diabetes Care. 2014;37(1):24–30.
20. Nordwall M, Bojestig M, Arnqvist HJ, Ludvigsson J. Declining incidence of severe retinopathy and persisting decrease of nephropathy in an unselected population of type 1 diabetes-the Linkoping Diabetes Complications Study. Diabetologia. 2004;47(7):1266–72.
21. Fullerton B, Jeitler K, Seitz M, Horvath K, Berghold A, Siebenhofer A. Intensive glucose control versus conventional glucose control for type 1 diabetes mellitus. Cochrane Database Syst Rev. 2014;2:CD009122.
22. Perkovic V, Heerspink HL, Chalmers J, Woodward M, Jun M, Li Q, et al. Intensive glucose control improves kidney outcomes in patients with type 2 diabetes. Kidney Int. 2013;83(3):517–23.
23. Ohkubo Y, Kishikawa H, Araki E, Miyata T, Isami S, Motoyoshi S, et al. Intensive insulin therapy prevents the progression of diabetic microvascular complications in Japanese patients with non-insulin-dependent diabetes mellitus: a randomized prospective 6-year study. Diabetes Res Clin Pract. 1995;28(2):103–17.
24. Brenner BM, Cooper ME, de Zeeuw D, Keane WF, Mitch WE, Parving HH, et al. Effects of losartan on renal and cardiovascular outcomes in patients with type 2 diabetes and nephropathy. N Engl J Med. 2001;345(12):861–9.
25. Lewis EJ, Hunsicker LG, Clarke WR, Berl T, Pohl MA, Lewis JB, et al. Renoprotective effect of the angiotensin-receptor antagonist irbesartan in patients with nephropathy due to type 2 diabetes. N Engl J Med. 2001;345(12):851–60.
26. Ravid M, Brosh D, Levi Z, Bar-Dayan Y, Ravid D, Rachmani R. Use of enalapril to attenuate decline in renal function in normotensive, normoalbuminuric patients with type 2 diabetes mellitus. A randomized, controlled trial. Ann Intern Med. 1998;128(12 Pt 1):982–8.

27. Wu JH, Foote C, Blomster J, Toyama T, Perkovic V, Sundstrom J, et al. Effects of sodium-glucose cotransporter-2 inhibitors on cardiovascular events, death, and major safety outcomes in adults with type 2 diabetes: a systematic review and meta-analysis. Lancet Diabetes Endocrinol. 2016;4(5):411–9.
28. Wanner C, Inzucchi SE, Lachin JM, Fitchett D, von Eynatten M, Mattheus M, et al. Empagliflozin and progression of kidney disease in type 2 diabetes. N Engl J Med. 2016;375(4):323–34.
29. Zinman B, Wanner C, Lachin JM, Fitchett D, Bluhmki E, Hantel S, et al. Empagliflozin, cardiovascular outcomes, and mortality in type 2 Diabetes. N Engl J Med. 2015;373(22):2117–28.
30. Perkovic V, Jardine MJ, Neal B, Bompoint S, Heerspink HJL, Charytan DM, et al. Canagliflozin and renal outcomes in type 2 diabetes and nephropathy. N Engl J Med. 2019;380(24):2295–306.
31. Edelman SV, Polonsky WH. Type 2 diabetes in the real world: the elusive nature of glycemic control. Diabetes Care. 2017;40(11):1425–32.
32. Yamanouchi M, Furuichi K, Hoshino J, Toyama T, Hara A, Shimizu M, et al. Nonproteinuric versus proteinuric phenotypes in diabetic kidney disease: a propensity score-matched analysis of a nationwide, biopsy-based cohort study. Diabetes Care. 2019;42(5):891–902.
33. Yokoyama H, Sone H, Oishi M, Kawai K, Fukumoto Y, Kobayashi M, et al. Prevalence of albuminuria and renal insufficiency and associated clinical factors in type 2 diabetes: the Japan Diabetes Clinical Data Management study (JDDM15). Nephrol Dial Transplant. 2009;24(4):1212–9.
34. Shimizu M, Furuichi K, Yokoyama H, Toyama T, Iwata Y, Sakai N, et al. Kidney lesions in diabetic patients with normoalbuminuric renal insufficiency. Clin Exp Nephrol. 2014;18(2):305–12.
35. Fioretto P, Mauer M, Brocco E, Velussi M, Frigato F, Muollo B, et al. Patterns of renal injury in NIDDM patients with microalbuminuria. Diabetologia. 1996;39(12):1569–76.
36. Klessens CQ, Woutman TD, Veraar KA, Zandbergen M, Valk EJ, Rotmans JI, et al. An autopsy study suggests that diabetic nephropathy is underdiagnosed. Kidney Int. 2016;90(1):149–56.
37. Furuichi K, Shimizu M, Yuzawa Y, Hara A, Toyama T, Kitamura H, et al. Clinicopathological analysis of biopsy-proven diabetic nephropathy based on the Japanese classification of diabetic nephropathy. Clin Exp Nephrol. 2017;22(3):570–82.
38. Furuichi K, Yuzawa Y, Shimizu M, Hara A, Toyama T, Kitamura H, et al. Nationwide multicentre kidney biopsy study of Japanese patients with type 2 diabetes. Nephrol Dial Transplant. 2017;33(1):138–48.
39. Hoshino J. A new pathological scoring system by the Japanese classification to predict renal outcome in diabetic nephropathy. PLoS One. 2017;13(2):e0190923.

Chapter 2
The Japanese Registries of Diabetic Nephropathy/Diabetic Kidney Disease

Miho Shimizu and Takashi Wada

2.1 Introduction

Chronic kidney disease (CKD) is diagnosed by the persistent presence of elevated urinary albumin excretion (albuminuria), low estimated glomerular filtration rate (eGFR), or other manifestations of kidney damage [1, 2]. Diabetic kidney disease (DKD), or CKD attributed to diabetes, occurs in 20–40% patients with diabetes [2–4]. Diabetic kidney disease is the leading cause of end-stage renal disease (ESRD) in Japan [5]. Additionally, the presence of CKD markedly increases cardiovascular risks in patients with diabetes [6].

Patient registries have great potential for providing data that describe the natural history, epidemiology, disease burden, treatments, and outcomes [7]. The Japan Renal Biopsy Registry (J-RBR) was started in 2007 and the Japan Kidney Disease Registry (J-KDR) was then started in 2009 by the Committee for Standardization of Renal Pathological Diagnosis and the Committee for the Kidney Disease Registry of the Japanese Society of Nephrology [8]. Clinical data including age, gender, and laboratory findings, in addition to histological diagnoses from renal biopsy, were electronically recorded at each institution and registered on the J-RBR/J-KDR web page via the Internet Data and Information Center of Medical Research system, which is part of the University hospital Medical Information Network. The latest

M. Shimizu (✉)
Department of Nephrology and Laboratory Medicine, Graduate School of Medical Sciences, Kanazawa University, Kanazawa, Japan

Health Service Center, Kanazawa University, Kanazawa, Japan
e-mail: mshimizu@staff.kanazawa-u.ac.jp

T. Wada
Department of Nephrology and Laboratory Medicine, Kanazawa University, Kanazawa, Japan

T. Wada et al. (eds.), *Diabetic Kidney Disease*,
https://doi.org/10.1007/978-981-15-9301-7_2

committee report by the J-RBR/J-KDR indicated that the prevalence of diabetic nephropathy in the J-RBR was 5.1% [9].

In addition to the J-RBR/J-KDR, the Japan Diabetic Nephropathy Cohort Study (JDNCS), a nationwide observational study for adult Japanese patients with type 2 diabetes and DKD (clinically suspected diabetic nephropathy), was initiated in 2009 [10, 11]. In the JDNCS, clinical data and urine samples are collected at least once a year during patient visits.

This review summarizes the clinical and laboratory findings concerning diabetic nephropathy/DKD using data registered in the J-RBR/J-KDR and the JDNCS.

2.2 Analysis of the J-RBR/J-KDR

Diabetic kidney disease is usually a clinical diagnosis made based on the presence of albuminuria and/or reduced eGFR in the absence of signs or symptoms of other primary causes of kidney damage [2]. The typical presentation of DKD is considered to include a long-standing duration of diabetes, retinopathy, albuminuria without hematuria, and gradually progressive kidney disease [2].

Of the 1591 patients with diabetes registered into the J-RBR from 2007 to 2013, 605 (38%) had a histological diagnosis of "diabetic nephropathy alone," whereas 986 (62%) had "nondiabetic renal disease (NDRD)." As shown in Table 2.1, patients

Table 2.1 Clinical characteristics of patients with diabetes who registered into the J-RBR by biopsy diagnosis

	Diabetic nephropathy alone		NDRD		*p*
	(*n* = 605)		(*n* = 986)		
Age (year)	59.5 ± 11.8	(*n* = 605)	61.8 ± 12.5	(*n* = 986)	<0.01
Male (%)	70.1	(*n* = 605)	65.4	(*n* = 986)	0.05
Body mass index (kg/m^2)	25.2 ± 4.2	(*n* = 580)	24.7 ± 4.4	(*n* = 959)	<0.01
Systolic blood pressure (mmHg)	144.2 ± 21.4	(*n* = 547)	135.3 ± 19.9	(*n* = 944)	<0.01
Diastolic blood pressure (mmHg)	78.8 ± 13.3	(*n* = 547)	77.4 ± 12.8	(*n* = 943)	<0.05
Antihypertensive agent use (%)	86.6	(*n* = 499)	73.8	(*n* = 866)	<0.01
Urinary protein excretion (g/day)	4.4 ± 3.5	(*n* = 441)	3.4 ± 3.4	(*n* = 616)	<0.01
UPCR (g/gCr)	6.0 ± 5.1	(*n* = 352)	4.3 ± 4.7	(*n* = 615)	<0.01
Nephrotic syndrome (%)	51.1	(*n* = 605)	33.1	(*n* = 986)	<0.01
Urine occult blood ≥ (+) (%)	49.9	(*n* = 605)	62.6	(*n* = 986)	<0.01
eGFR (mL/min/1.73 m^2)	48.1 ± 24.0	(*n* = 603)	51.5 ± 26.9	(*n* = 981)	<0.01
Serum total protein (g/dL)	6.2 ± 1.1	(*n* = 599)	6.4 ± 1.2	(*n* = 971)	<0.01
Serum albumin (g/dL)	3.1 ± 0.9	(*n* = 597)	3.2 ± 1.0	(*n* = 966)	<0.01
Serum total cholesterol (mg/dL)	222.7 ± 76.5	(*n* = 577)	227.7 ± 91.5	(*n* = 936)	0.95
Hemoglobin A1c (%)	7.2 ± 1.7	(*n* = 578)	6.9 ± 1.1	(*n* = 888)	<0.05

Abbreviations: *eGFR* estimated glomerular filtration rate, *NDRD* nondiabetic renal disease, *UPCR* urinary protein-to-creatinine ratio

Table 2.2 Association of clinical predictors and biopsy findings of diabetic nephropathy alone in the J-RBR

	HR	(95% CI)	*p*
Antihypertensive agent use (+)	2.166	(1.53–3.07)	<0.01
Dipstick proteinuria (≥2+)	2.054	(1.45–2.90)	<0.01
Dipstick hematuria (−)	1.861	(1.43–2.43)	<0.01
Serum total protein (−1 g/dL)	1.263	(1.11–1.44)	<0.01
Hemoglobin A1c (+1 %)	1.235	(1.12–1.37)	<0.01
Age (−1 year)	1.027	(1.02–1.04)	<0.01
Mean blood pressure (+1 mmHg)	1.012	(1.00–1.02)	<0.01
eGFR (−1 mL/min/1.73 m^2)	1.009	(1.00–1.01)	<0.01
Total cholesterol (−1 mg/dL)	1.004	(1.00–1.01)	<0.01

Abbreviations: *CI* confidence intervals, *eGFR* estimated glomerular filtration rate, *HR* hazard ratio

with "diabetic nephropathy alone" were significantly younger; had higher levels of body mass index, systolic and diastolic blood pressure, urinary protein excretion, and hemoglobin A1c; higher prevalence of antihypertensive agent use and nephrotic syndrome; lower levels of eGFR, serum total protein, and serum albumin; and lower prevalence of hematuria than patients with "NDRD." By multivariate logistic regression analysis, antihypertensive agent use, severe proteinuria (dipstick proteinuria ≥2+), absence of hematuria, low serum total protein, high hemoglobin A1c, young age, high mean blood pressure, low eGFR, and low total cholesterol were found to be significantly associated with "diabetic nephropathy alone" (Table 2.2).

2.3 Analysis of the JDNCS

2.3.1 Clinical Characteristics at Enrollment

Glomerular filtration rate and albuminuria are clinical markers of diabetic nephropathy [2–4]. Clinical variables at enrollment were compared among subgroups stratified by eGFR and albuminuria in 567 patients whose eGFR and albuminuria data at enrollment were available from July 2009 to October 2017 in the JDNCS (Table 2.3). The median total cohort age was 67 years [interquartile range (IQR), 59–73 years], and 66.3% patients were male. Variables associated with low eGFR (<60 mL/min/1.73 m^2), regardless of albuminuria, were advanced age, high prevalence of retinopathy and renin-angiotensin system (RAS) inhibitor use, and low levels of hemoglobin A1c, serum total cholesterol, and hemoglobin. On the other hand, variables associated with albuminuria, regardless of eGFR category, were high level of serum triglyceride and high prevalence of retinopathy and RAS inhibitor use.

Microalbuminuria has been considered the first clinical sign of diabetic nephropathy. However, recent studies demonstrated that reduced eGFR without albuminuria is frequently reported in patients with type 1 and 2 diabetes [2–4]. The reported

Table 2.3 Clinical characteristics at enrollment stratified by initial eGFR and albuminuria categories in the JDNCS

	All	Normoalbuminuria			Micro-/macroalbuminuria			eGFR ≥ 60	eGFR < 60
		eGFR ≥ 60	eGFR < 60	*p* for eGFR ≥ 60 vs. eGFR < 60	eGFR ≥ 60	eGFR < 60	*p* for eGFR ≥ 60 vs. eGFR < 60	*p* for Normo vs. Micro-/macroalbuminuria	*p* for Normo vs. Micro-/macroalbuminuria
Total N	567	162	53		104	248			
Age (years)	67.0 (59.0–73.0)	64.0 (57.0–70.0)	70.0 (65.0–75.0)	<0.01	63.0 (55.0–72.0)	68.5 (61.3–74.0)	<0.01	0.99	0.10
Male (%)	66.3	58.6	49.1	0.22	70.2	73.4	0.54	0.06	<0.01
Serum creatinine (mg/dL)	0.9 (0.7–1.8)	0.7 (0.6–0.8)	1.1 (0.9–1.2)	<0.01	0.72 (0.61–0.84)	2.1 (1.3–4.1)	<0.01	0.17	<0.01
eGFR (mL/min/1.73 m^2)	57.7 (27.8–75.9)	76.7 (68.6–92.2)	48.3 (41.3–55.1)	<0.01	77.3 (66.8–91.0)	24.7 (11.5–40.1)	<0.01	0.61	<0.01
Diabetes duration (years)	12.0 (7.0–20.0)	10.0 (5.0–17.0)	11.0 (5.0–20.0)	0.16	10.0 (5.0–20/0)	14.5 (9.0–23.0)	<0.01	0.62	0.11
Diabetic retinopathy (%)	50.6	24.3	48.0	<0.01	45.4	69.0	<0.01	<0.01	<0.01
Hemoglobin A1c (%)	7.0 (6.4–7.8)	7.3 (6.8–8.0)	6.7 (6.4–7.5)	<0.01	7.3 (6.6–8.8)	6.6 (6.1–7.4)	<0.01	0.77	0.43
Oral hypoglycemic agents (%)	66.1	71.5	80.8	0.19	67.0	59.0	0.16	0.44	<0.01
Insulin (%)	42.7	38.4	38.5	0.99	43.1	46.1	0.61	0.44	0.31

Systolic blood pressure (mmHg)	130.0 (118.0–142.0)	124.0 (116.0–138.0)	126.0 (116.0–134.5)	0.62	128.0 (114.0–141.0)	134.0 (122.0–150.0)	<0.05	0.22	<0.01
Diastolic blood pressure (mmHg)	72.0 (65.0–80.0)	74.0 (67.0–82.0)	70.0 (59.0–77.0)	<0.01	74.0 (67.0–81.0)	72.0 (64.0–80.0)	0.23	0.67	<0.05
Use of RAS inhibitors (%)	65.9	42.1	65.4	<0.01	66.0	81.3	<0.01	<0.01	<0.05
Total cholesterol (mg/dL)	179.0 (152.0–203.0)	185.5 (164.3–208.8)	168.0 (154.0–192.5)	<0.05	187.0 (159.5–209.5)	172.0 (140.0–200.0)	<0.05	0.99	0.84
HDL-cholesterol (mg/dL)	46.0 (38.0–57.0)	51.5 (42.3–61.0)	48.0 (39.3–61.0)	0.27	46.0 (38.0–55.0)	43.0 (36.0–55.0)	0.34	<0.01	0.07
Triglyceride (mg/dL)	120.0 (82.8–176.0)	111.0 (74.0–175.5)	95.0 (75.5–141.0)	0.38	139.0 (98.3–195.8)	121.5 (89.0–175.8)	0.07	<0.01	<0.05
Use of statins (%)	46.1	42.1	48.1	0.45	40.8	50.4	0.10	0.83	0.76
Body mass index (kg/m^2)	24.4 (21.9–27.0)	24.3 (22.4–27.0)	24.7 (21.4–27.5)	0.85	25.2 (21.9–28.7)	24.1 (21.8–26.8)	0.15	0.42	0.54
Hemoglobin (mg/dL)	12.6 (10.9–13.9)	13.7 (12.7–14.6)	11.9 (11.1–13.1)	<0.01	13.6 (12.3–14.6)	11.3 (9.7–12.6)	<0.01	0.49	<0.01
Current smoking (%)	23.7	23.7	14.0	0.15	27.7	24.2	0.51	0.49	0.12

Abbreviations: *eGFR* estimated glomerular filtration rate, *HDL* high-density lipoprotein, *RAS* renin-angiotensin system

clinical characteristics of diabetic patients with normoalbuminuric renal insufficiency included a shorter diabetes duration, higher levels of hemoglobin and high-density lipoprotein (HDL) cholesterol, higher prevalence of females, lower levels of hemoglobin A1c and triglyceride, and lower prevalence of hypertension, smoking, retinopathy, neuropathy, previous cardiovascular disease, and antihypertensive agent use including RAS inhibitors than patients with albuminuric renal insufficiency [12–14]. Additionally, compared with patients with normoalbuminuric-preserved renal function, patients with normoalbuminuric renal insufficiency were older and had higher level of insulin resistance and higher prevalence of female, nonsmoker, hypertension, dyslipidemia, metabolic syndrome, and previous cardiovascular diseases [12, 15]. In the JDNCS, patients with normoalbuminuria and low eGFR had significantly higher levels of eGFR and hemoglobin; higher prevalence of female and oral hypoglycemic agent use; lower levels of serum creatinine, systolic and diastolic blood pressure, and triglyceride; and lower prevalence of retinopathy and RAS inhibitor use than patients with micro-/macroalbuminuria and low eGFR (Table 2.3). Furthermore, when compared with patients with normoalbuminuria and preserved eGFR, patients with normoalbuminuria and low eGFR were significantly older and had higher prevalence of retinopathy and RAS inhibitor use and lower levels of hemoglobin A1c, diastolic blood pressure, total cholesterol, and hemoglobin (Table 2.3).

Although the pathogenesis of normoalbuminuric renal insufficiency in patients with diabetes remains inconclusive, several studies, including our prior studies that evaluated 260 Japanese patients with type 2 diabetes and biopsy-proven diabetic nephropathy, revealed that disproportionately advanced tubulointerstitial and vascular lesions, despite minor diabetic glomerular lesions, which denote the presence of diabetic kidney lesions as well as nephrosclerosis, were likely to be related to the development of normoalbuminuric renal insufficiency in patients with type 2 diabetes [16–18].

2.3.2 Clinical Variables at Enrollment Associated with Outcomes

During a median follow-up of 6 years (IQR, 1.8–7 years), a total of 89 cases of ESRD (requirement of dialysis), 59 cardiovascular events (cardiovascular death, nonfatal myocardial infarction, coronary interventions, nonfatal stroke, or peripheral arterial disease), and 32 deaths were observed. The results of a multivariate Cox proportional hazards regression analysis are shown in Table 2.4. Macroalbuminuria (or severe proteinuria defined as urinary protein-to-creatinine (UPCR) $\geq$ 0.5 g/gCr), eGFR < 60 mL/min/1.73 m^2, male gender, systolic blood pressure $\geq$ 140 mmHg and/or diastolic blood pressure $\geq$ 90 mmHg, low hemoglobin, and young age were independent risk factors for ESRD. Male gender, low hemoglobin, high hemoglobin A1c, advanced age, and high total cholesterol were independent risk factors for

Table 2.4 Variables at enrollment associated with ESRD, cardiovascular events, and all-cause mortality in the JDNCS

Variables	HR	(95% CI)	p
ESRD			
Macroalbuminuria (severe proteinuria)	10.60	(4.055–27.682)	<0.01
eGFR < 60 mL/min/1.73 m^2	5.81	(1.684–20.024)	<0.01
Male gender	2.48	(1.300–4.740)	<0.01
Systolic blood pressure ≥ 140 mm Hg and/or diastolic blood pressure ≥ 90 mmHg	2.25	(1.390–3.642)	<0.01
Hemoglobin (−1 g/dL)	1.25	(1.104–1.420)	<0.01
Age (−1 year)	1.03	(1.003–1.047)	<0.05
Cardiovascular events			
Male gender	4.04	(1.870–8.745)	<0.01
Hemoglobin (−1 g/dL)	1.33	(1.155–1.533)	<0.01
Hemoglobin A1c (+1 %)	1.24	(1.049–1.460)	<0.05
Age (+1 year)	1.04	(1.006–1.065)	<0.05
Total cholesterol (+1 mg/dL)	1.01	(1.001–1.013)	<0.05
All-cause mortality			
Macroalbuminuria (severe proteinuria)	5.34	(2.222–12.851)	<0.01
Age (+1 year)	1.09	(1.043–1.137)	<0.01

Hazard ratio was adjusted for age, gender, eGFR <60 mL/min/1.73 m^2, macroalbuminuria, hemoglobin A1c, systolic blood pressure, use of renin-angiotensin system inhibitors, total cholesterol, body mass index, and hemoglobin
Abbreviations: *CI* confidence intervals, *eGFR* estimated glomerular filtration rate, *ESRD* end-stage renal disease, *HR* hazard ratio

cardiovascular events. Macroalbuminuria (or severe proteinuria) and advanced age were independent risk factors for all-cause mortality.

Although the outcomes of patients with diabetes and normoalbuminuric renal insufficiency also remain controversial, our previous study revealed that the cumulative incidence of renal composite events (requirement of dialysis, or 50% decline in eGFR from baseline), cardiovascular events (cardiovascular death, nonfatal myocardial infarction, coronary interventions, and nonfatal stroke), and all-cause mortality in patients with normoalbuminuria was not significantly different among eGFR categories [16, 17]. In the JDNCS, it was impossible to examine the survival analysis of patients with normoalbuminuria because of insufficient number of events.

2.3.3 Transition in eGFR and UACR Categories

The transition in eGFR and urinary albumin-to-creatinine ratio (UACR) categories during the follow-up were explored based on the new CKD classification [1]. This analysis was conducted in 456 patients whose data for eGFR and UACR were available between July 2007 and December 2015 in the JDNCS. The median follow-up period was 4.2 years (IQR, 2.0–5.0 years). Compared with the eGFR category at enrollment, 137 of 393 patients (34.9%) with eGFR $\geq$ 15 mL/min/1.73 m^2 (categories G1–4) progressed to a lower eGFR category, and 32 of 388 patients (8.2%) with eGFR < 90 mL/min/1.73 m^2 (categories G2–5) regressed to a higher eGFR category (Fig. 2.1a). Examination of UACR at enrollment revealed that 34 of 151 patients (22.5%) with normoalbuminuria (<30 mg/gCr [category A1]) and 15 of 79 patients (19.0%) with microalbuminuria ($\geq$30 and <300 mg/gCr [category A2]) progressed to a higher ACR category. Contrarily, 19 of 79 patients (24.1%) with microalbuminuria (A2) and 20 of 132 patients (15.2%) with macroalbuminuria ($\geq$300 mg/gCr [category A3]) regressed to a lower ACR category (Fig. 2.1b).

2.3.4 Percentage Changes in eGFR and ESRD

There is an increased interest in surrogate endpoints for clinical CKD trials. The established hard endpoints of serum creatinine doubling, renal replacement therapy, and renal death are late events, requiring long follow-up periods and large sample sizes. A series of meta-analyses of clinical trials and observational studies have revealed a relationship between lesser declines than a halving in eGFR and ESRD [19–24]. However, these large studies were conducted across several CKD causes.

In the JDNCS, the association of ESRD with percentage change in eGFR during 1- and 2-year baseline periods was evaluated among four categories based on percentage changes in eGFR: $\leq$−50%, >−50 to−30%, >−30 to 0%, and >0%. This analysis was applied to patients having macroalbuminuria at enrollment and at least

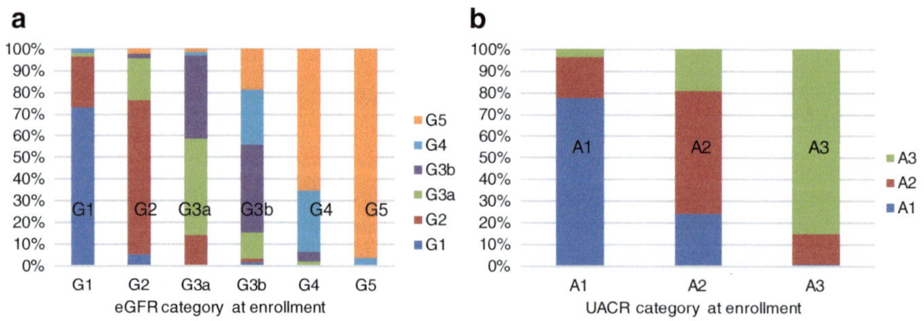

Fig. 2.1 Proportion of patients who transited in (**a**) eGFR and (**b**) UACR categories during the follow-up in the JDNCS

two eGFR measurements during a baseline period before reaching ESRD. In the 1-year baseline period analysis, cumulative ESRD incidence in macroalbuminuric patients with ≤−50% change was higher than in those with >−50 to−30% change ($p < 0.05$), >−30 to 0% change ($p < 0.01$), and >0% change ($p < 0.01$) (Fig. 2.2a). Additionally, the cumulative ESRD incidence in macroalbuminuric patients with changes >−50 to−30% was also higher than in those with>−30 to 0% change ($p < 0.05$) and >0% change ($p < 0.01$) (Fig. 2.2a). In the 2-year baseline period analysis, the cumulative ESRD incidence in macroalbuminuric patients with ≤−50% change was higher than those in patients with −30 to 0% change ($p < 0.01$) and >0% change ($p < 0.01$) (Fig. 2.2b). The cumulative ESRD incidence in macroalbuminuric patients with changes >−50 to −30% was also higher than in those with >−30 to 0% change ($p < 0.05$) and >0% change ($p < 0.05$) (Fig. 2.2b). In the 2-year analysis, there was no difference in the cumulative ESRD incidence between patients with changes ≤−50 and >−50 to −30% (Fig. 2.2b). Compared with patients with stable eGFR (>−30 to 0% change), the risk of ESRD in patients with ≤−50% change increased at the 1-year analysis [crude HR 9.16 (95% CI 3.02–27.77; $p < 0.01$); adjusted HR 16.80 (95% CI 2.19–128.88; $p < 0.01$)] and the 2-year analysis [crude HR 13.31 (95% CI 2.44–72.66; $p < 0.01$); adjusted HR 45.73 (95% CI 4.90–426.34; $p < 0.01$)] (Table 2.5). Although not as much as in patients with ≤−50% change, the risk of ESRD in patients with >−50 to–30% change was also

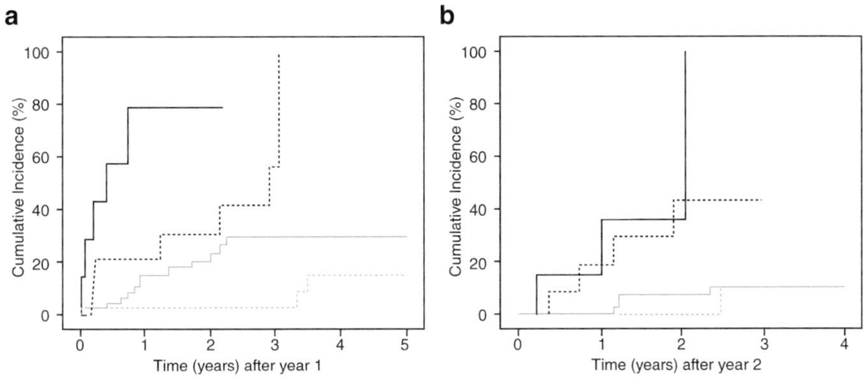

Fig. 2.2 Cumulative incidence of ESRD compared among groups stratified by percentage changes in eGFR during (**a**) 1-year and (**b**) 2-year baseline periods in the JDNCS. (**a**) Black solid line, ≤−50% change ($n = 7$); black dotted line, >−50 to −30% change ($n = 21$); gray solid line, >−30 to 0% change ($n = 168$); gray dotted line, >0% change ($n = 142$) during 1-year baseline period. Cumulative incidence of ESRD in patients with ≤−50% change in eGFR was significantly higher than in those with >−50 to −30% change ($p < 0.05$), >−30 to 0% change ($p < 0.01$), and >0% change ($p < 0.01$). Cumulative incidence of ESRD in patients with >−50 to −30% change was significantly higher than in those with >−30 to 0% change ($p < 0.05$) and >0% change ($p < 0.01$). (**b**) Black solid line, ≤−50% change ($n = 7$); black dotted line, >−50 to −30% change ($n = 16$); gray solid line, >−30 to 0% change ($n = 155$); gray dotted line, >0% change ($n = 107$) during 2-year baseline period. Cumulative incidence of ESRD in patients with ≤−50% change was significantly higher than those in patients with −30 to 0% change ($p < 0.01$) and >0% change ($p < 0.01$). Cumulative incidence of ESRD in patients with >−50 to −30% change was significantly higher than in those with >−30 to 0% change ($p < 0.05$) and >0% change ($p < 0.05$). There was no difference between ≤−50% change and >−50 to −30% change

Table 2.5 Crude and adjusted HR of percentage change in eGFR, initial eGFR, and initial UPCR on ESRD in 1-year and 2-year analyses in the JDNCS

	1-year baseline period						2-year baseline period					
Predictor	Univariate			Multivariate			Univariate			Multivariate		
	HR	(95% CI)	*p*	HR	(95% CI)	*p*	HR	(95% CI)	*p*	HR	(95% CI)	*p*
Percentage change in eGFR												
>0%	0.36	(0.10–1.26)	0.11	0.46	(0.13–1.69)	0.24	0.79	(0.08–7.59)	0.84	1.18	(0.11–12.26)	0.89
<−30 to 0%	1	(Reference)		1	(Reference)		1	(Reference)		1	(Reference)	
<−50 to −30%	2.87	(1.10–7.47)	<0.05	3.89	(1.17–12.92)	<0.05	6.20	(1.37–28.01)	<0.05	15.55	(1.76–137.18)	<0.05
≤−50%	9.16	(3.02–27.77)	<0.01	16.80	(2.19–128.88)	<0.01	13.31	(2.44–72.66)	<0.01	45.73	(4.90–426.34)	<0.01
Initial eGFR (−1 mL/min/1.73 m^2)	1.09	(1.05–1.13)	<0.01	1.15	(1.08–1.22)	<0.01	1.06	(1.02–1.11)	<0.01	1.12	(1.03–1.21)	<0.01
Initial UPCR (+1 g/gCr)	1.31	(1.17–1.46)	<0.01	0.89	(0.74–1.08)	0.23	1.23	(0.98–1.55)	0.07	0.79	(0.56–1.10)	0.16

Hazard ratio was adjusted for age, gender, hemoglobin A1c, systolic blood pressure, use of renin-angiotensin system inhibitors, total cholesterol, body mass index, and hemoglobin in a multivariate analysis

Abbreviations: *CI* confidence intervals, *eGFR* estimated glomerular filtration rate, *ESRD* end-stage renal disease, *HR* hazard ratio, *UPCR* urinary protein-to-creatinine ratio

increased at the 1-year analysis [crude HR 2.87 (95% CI 1.10–7.47; $p < 0.05$); adjusted HR 3.89 (95% CI 1.17–12.92; $p < 0.05$)] and the 2-year analysis [crude HR 6.20 (95% CI 1.37–28.01; $p < 0.05$); adjusted HR 15.55 (95% CI 1.76–137.18; $p < 0.05$)] (Table 2.5). These findings are in line with other recent reports showing the utility of eGFR slope in type 2 diabetes as a surrogate endpoint for the renal outcome [25, 26].

2.3.5 *Remission of Macroalbuminuria and ESRD*

Recent RCT meta-analyses provided empirical evidence for using changes in albuminuria as a surrogate marker for ESRD [27]. Several observational studies, in addition to interventional trials, have shown that remission of macroalbuminuria and/or reduction in albuminuria predicts better renal outcomes in patients with diabetes and overt nephropathy [28–32]. In the JDNCS, the association of ESRD with remission of macroalbuminuria during the 1- and 2-year baseline periods was also evaluated. This analysis was applied to patients having macroalbuminuria at enrollment and at least two UACR (or UPCR) measurements during a baseline period before reaching ESRD. Remission was defined as transition from macroalbuminuria to normo-/microalbuminuria. Macroalbuminuric patients with remission had lower cumulative ESRD incidences than patients with no remission at the 1-year ($p < 0.05$, Fig. 2.3a) and 2-year analysis ($p < 0.01$, Fig. 2.3b). However, remission was not a determinant for ESRD independent of initial eGFR and UPCR by multivariate analysis (Table 2.6). Our results may be explained by the irreversibility of kidney

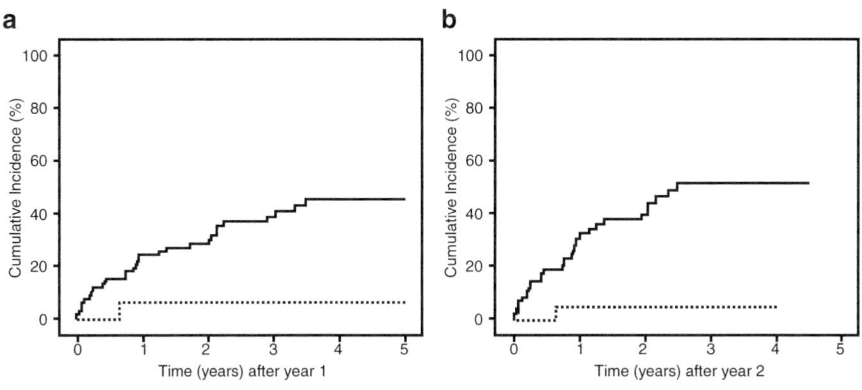

Fig. 2.3 Cumulative incidence of ESRD compared among groups with or without remission of macroalbuminuria during (**a**) 1-year and (**b**) 2-year baseline periods in the JDNCS. (**a**) Solid line, without remission group ($n = 94$); dotted line, with remission group ($n = 18$) after year 1. Cumulative incidence of ESRD in patients with remission was significantly lower than in those without remission ($p < 0.05$). (**b**) Solid line, without remission group ($n = 90$); dotted line, with remission group ($n = 23$) after year 2. Cumulative incidence of ESRD in patients with remission was significantly lower than in those without remission ($p < 0.01$)

Table 2.6 Crude and adjusted HR of remission of macroalbuminuria, initial eGFR, and initial UPCR on ESRD in 1-year and 2-year analyses in the JDNCS

	1-year baseline period						2-year baseline period					
Predictor	Univariate			Multivariate			Univariate			Multivariate		
	HR	(95% CI)	*p*	HR	(95% CI)	*p*	HR	(95% CI)	*p*	HR	(95% CI)	*p*
Remission of macroalbuminuria												
(−)	1	(Reference)		1	(Reference)		1	(Reference)		1	(Reference)	
(+)	0.14	(0.02–1.01)	0.05	0.23	(0.03–1.78)	0.16	0.09	(0.01–0.64)	<0.05	0.31	(0.04–2.39)	0.26
Initial eGFR (−1 mL/min/1.73 m^2)	1.08	(1.04–1.11)	<0.01	1.07	(1.04–1.11)	<0.01	1.07	(1.04–1.11)	<0.01	1.07	(1.04–1.11)	<0.01
Initial UPCR (+1 g/gCr)	1.28	(1.17–1.41)	<0.01	1.19	(1.06–1.32)	<0.01	1.29	(1.18–1.42)	<0.01	1.20	(1.07–1.33)	<0.01

Hazard ratio was adjusted for age, gender, hemoglobin A1c, systolic blood pressure, use of renin-angiotensin system inhibitors, total cholesterol, body mass index, and hemoglobin in a multivariate analysis

Abbreviations: *CI* confidence intervals, *eGFR* estimated glomerular filtration rate, *ESRD* end-stage renal disease, *HR* hazard ratio, *UPCR* urinary protein-to-creatinine ratio

lesions. In our prior study regarding biopsy-proven diabetic nephropathy with type 2 diabetes, the characteristic pathological lesions (glomerular lesions, interstitial fibrosis and tubular atrophy, and arteriosclerosis) as well as clinical factors including macroalbuminuria and reduced eGFR were independent determinants of renal composite events [16]. Analyses addressing the relationships between pathological information related to changes in albuminuria and renal outcomes would advance our understanding of albuminuria as a surrogate endpoint for determining outcomes in patients with diabetic nephropathy. Additionally, several studies have reported a high relapse rate in patients with diabetes who achieved remission of macroalbuminuria [29, 33].

2.4 Conclusion

The J-RBR/J-KDR and the JDCNS developed by the Japanese Society of Nephrology provide nationwide cohort data for epidemiological studies of diabetic nephropathy/DKD. Additionally, the Japanese Society of Nephrology and the Japan Association for Medical Informatics have constructed a comprehensive clinical database of CKD patients called the Japan Chronic Kidney Disease Database (J-CKD-DB) based on advanced electronic health record systems to automatically extract data using the Standardized Structured Medical Information eXchange (SS-MIX2) [34]. These registries included patients who received treatment according to national guidelines by nephrologist, supporting high external validity and generalizability to other population with type 2 diabetes.

Acknowledgments This study was supported in part by a Grant-in-Aid for Diabetic Nephropathy Research from the Ministry of Health, Labour and Welfare of Japan, a Grant-in-Aid for Diabetic Nephropathy and Nephrosclerosis Research from the Ministry of Health, Labour and Welfare of Japan, and a Grant-in-Aid for Practical Research Project for Renal Diseases from the Japan Agency for Medical Research and Development (JP17ek0310003). This study was also supported in part by JSPS KAKENHI (17K08979) (M.S.) and Grant from the Kidney Foundation, Japan (JKFB19–8) (M.S.).

Disclosure None declared.

References

1. Levey AS, de Jong PE, Coresh J, El Nahas M, Astor BC, Matsushita K, et al. The definition, classification, and prognosis of chronic kidney disease: a KDIGO Controversies Conference report. Kidney Int. 2011;80:17–28.
2. American Diabetes Association. Microvascular complications and foot care: standards of medical care in diabetes-2018. Diabetes Care. 2018;41(Suppl 1):S105–18.
3. Tuttle KR, Bakris GL, Bilous RW, Chiang JL, de Boer IH, Goldstein-Fuchs J, et al. Diabetic kidney disease: a report from an ADA Consensus Conference. Diabetes Care. 2014;37:2864–83.

4. Afkarian M, Zelnick LR, Hall YN, Heagerty PJ, Tuttle K, Weiss NS, et al. Clinical manifestations of kidney disease among US adults with diabetes, 1988–2014. JAMA. 2016;316:602–10.
5. Masakane I, Nakai S, Ogata S, Kimata N, Hanafusa N, Hamano T, et al. An overview of regular dialysis treatment in Japan (As of 31 December 2013). Ther Apher Dial. 2015;19:540–74.
6. Fox CS, Matsushita K, Woodward M, Bilo HJ, Chalmers J, Heerspink HJ, et al. Associations of kidney disease measures with mortality and end-stage renal disease in individuals with and without diabetes: a meta-analysis. Lancet. 2012;380:1662–73.
7. Liu FX, Rutherford P, Smoyer-Tomic K, Prichard S, Laplante S. A global overview of renal registries: a systematic review. BMC Nephrol. 2015;16:31. https://doi.org/10.1186/s12882-015-0028-2.
8. Sugiyama H, Yokoyama H, Sato H, Saito T, Kohda Y, Nishi S, et al. Japan Renal Biopsy Registry: the first nationwide, web-based, and prospective registry system of renal biopsies in Japan. Clin Exp Nephrol. 2011;15:493–503.
9. Sugiyama H, Yokoyama H, Sato H, Saito T, Kohda Y, Nishi S, et al. Japan renal biopsy registry and Japan kidney disease registry: Committee report for 2009 and 2010. Clin Exp Nephrol. 2013;17:155–73.
10. Furuichi K, Shimizu M, Toyama T, Koya D, Koshino Y, Abe H, et al. Japan Diabetic Nephropathy Cohort Study: study design, methods, and implementation. Clin Exp Nephrol. 2013;17:819–26.
11. Shimizu M, Furuichi K, Toyama T, Funamoto T, Kitajima S, Hara A, et al. Decline in estimated glomerular filtration rate is associated with risk of end-stage renal disease in type 2 diabetes with macroalbuminuria: an observational study from JDNCS. Clin Exp Nephrol. 2017;22(2):377–87. https://doi.org/10.1007/s10157-017-1467-9.
12. Afghahi H, Cederholm J, Eliasson B, Zethelius B, Gudbjörnsdottir S, Hadimeri H, et al. Risk factors for the development of albuminuria and renal impairment in type 2 diabetes—the Swedish National Diabetes Register (NDR). Nephrol Dial Transplant. 2011;26:1236–43.
13. Fioretto P, Mauer M, Brocco E, Velussi M, Frigato F, Muollo B, et al. Patterns of renal injury in NIDDM patients with microalbuminuria. Diabetologia. 1996;39:1569–76.
14. Fioretto P, Caramori ML, Mauer M. The kidney in diabetes: dynamic pathways of injury and repair. The Camillo Golgi Lecture 2007. Diabetologia. 2008;51:1347–55.
15. Gambara V, Mecca G, Remuzzi G, Bertani T. Heterogeneous nature of renal lesions in type II diabetes. J Am Soc Nephrol. 1993;3:1458–66.
16. Shimizu M, Furuichi K, Toyama T, Kitajima S, Hara A, Kitagawa K, et al. Long-term outcomes of Japanese type 2 diabetic patients with biopsy-proven diabetic nephropathy. Diabetes Care. 2013;36:3655–62.
17. Shimizu M, Furuichi K, Yokoyama H, Toyama T, Sakai N, Iwata Y, et al. Kidney lesions in diabetic patients with normoalbuminuric renal insufficiency. Clin Exp Nephrol. 2014;18:305–12.
18. Ekinci EI, Jerums G, Skene A, Crammer P, Power D, Cheong KY, et al. Renal structure in normoalbuminuric and albuminuric patients with type 2 diabetes and impaired renal function. Diabetes Care. 2013;36:3620–6.
19. Coresh J, Turin TC, Matsushita K, Sang Y, Ballew SH, Appel LJ, et al. Decline in estimated glomerular filtration rate and subsequent risk of end-stage renal disease and mortality. JAMA. 2014;311:2518–31.
20. Levey AS, Inker LA, Matsushita K, Greene T, Willis K, Lewis E, et al. GFR decline as an end point for clinical trials in CKD: a scientific workshop sponsored by the National Kidney Foundation and the US Food and Drug Administration. Am J Kidney Dis. 2014;64:821–35.
21. Inker LA, Lambers Heerspink HJ, Mondal H, Schmid CH, Tighiouart H, Noubary F, et al. GFR decline as an alternative end point to kidney failure in clinical trials: a meta-analysis of treatment effects from 37 randomized trials. Am J Kidney Dis. 2014;64:848–59.
22. Lambers Heerspink HJ, Tighiouart H, Sang Y, Ballew S, Mondal H, Matsushita K, et al. GFR decline and subsequent risk of established kidney outcomes: a meta-analysis of 37 randomized controlled trials. Am J Kidney Dis. 2014;64:860–6.

23. Greene T, Teng CC, Inker LA, Redd A, Ying J, Woodward M, et al. Utility and validity of estimated GFR based surrogate time-to-event end points in CKD: a simulation study. Am J Kidney Dis. 2014;64:867–79.
24. Matsushita K, Chen J, Sang Y, Ballew SH, Shimazaki R, Fukagawa M, et al. Risk of end-stage renal disease in Japanese patients with chronic kidney disease increases proportionately to decline in estimated glomerular filtration rate. Kidney Int. 2016;90:1109–14.
25. Oshima M, Toyama T, Haneda M, Furuichi K, Babazono T, Yokoyama H, et al. Estimated glomerular filtration rate decline and risk of end-stage renal disease in type 2 diabetes. PLoS One. 2018;13:e0201535.
26. Oshima M, Jun M, Ohkuma T, Toyama T, Wada T, Cooper ME, et al. The relationship between eGFR slope and subsequent risk of vascular outcomes and all-cause mortality in type 2 diabetes: the ADVANCE-ON study. Diabetologia. 2019;62:1988–97.
27. Heerspink HJ, Kröpelin TF, Hoekman J, de Zeeuw D. Reducing Albuminuria as Surrogate Endpoint (REASSURE) Consortium. Drug-induced reduction in albuminuria is associated with subsequent renoprotection: a meta-analysis. J Am Soc Nephrol. 2015;26:2055–64.
28. de Boer IH, Afkarian M, Rue TC, Cleary PA, Lachin JM, Molitch ME, et al. Renal outcomes in patients with type 1 diabetes and macroalbuminuria. J Am Soc Nephrol. 2014;25:2342–50.
29. Yokoyama H, Araki S, Honjo J, Okizaki S, Yamada D, Shudo R, et al. Association between remission of macroalbuminuria and preservation of renal function in patients with type 2 diabetes with overt proteinuria. Diabetes Care. 2013;36:3227–33.
30. Imai E, Haneda M, Chan JC, Yamasaki T, Kobayashi F, Ito S, et al. Reduction and residual proteinuria are therapeutic targets in type 2 diabetes with overt nephropathy: a post hoc analysis (ORIENT-proteinuria). Nephrol Dial Transplant. 2013;28:2526–34.
31. de Zeeuw D, Remuzzi G, Parving HH, Keane WF, Zhang Z, Shahinfar S, et al. Proteinuria, a target for renoprotection in patients with type 2 diabetic nephropathy: lessons from RENAAL. Kidney Int. 2004;65:2309–20.
32. Atkins RC, Briganti EM, Lewis JB, Hunsicker LG, Braden G, Champion de Crespigny PJ, et al. Proteinuria reduction and progression to renal failure in patients with type 2 diabetes mellitus and overt nephropathy. Am J Kidney Dis. 2005;45:281–7.
33. Hovind P, Rossing P, Tarnow L, Toft H, Parving J, Parving HH. Remission of nephrotic-range albuminuria in type 1 diabetic patients. Diabetes Care. 2001;24:1972–7.
34. Nakagawa N, Sofue T, Kanda E, Nagasu H, Matsushita K, Nangaku M, et al. J-CKD-DB: a nationwide multicentre electronic health record-based chronic kidney disease database in Japan. Sci Rep. 2020;10:7351.

Chapter 3
Diabetic Kidney Disease and Cardiovascular Disease

Kumiko Muta, Yoko Obata, and Tomoya Nishino

3.1 Introduction

It has been known that diabetes is associated with a high risk of cardiovascular disease (CVD) [1]. The hazard ratio (HR) among individuals with diabetes as compared to those without diabetes was 2.32 for deaths from vascular causes after adjustment for baseline age, sex, smoking status, and body mass index in an individual participant meta-analysis of data over 1.1 million participants from 104 cohorts in predominantly Western populations by the independent academic coordinating center of the Emerging Risk Factors Collaboration [2]. It has been reported that CVD is also frequently associated with chronic kidney disease (CKD) [3]. In a study involving patients with CKD stage 3 (estimated glomerular filtration rate (eGFR) between 30 and 59 mL/min/1.73 m^2), the number of deaths was more than that from end-stage renal disease (ESRD) [4]. Based on these reports, it is naturally thought that diabetic kidney disease (DKD), which refers to kidney disease that is specific to diabetes, may also be associated with CVD. For the risk of CVD, in both diabetes and CKD, there are some referenced studies regarding the impact of kidney disease on mortality in diabetic patients. The Finnish Diabetic Nephropathy Study was a nationwide prospective study of 4201 adults with type 1 diabetes [5]. In this study, during a median 7 years of follow-up, overall mortality rate was 3.6 times higher than that in the age- and sex-matched general population, and the presence and severity of CKD were the major predictors of all-cause mortality [5]. In the Pittsburgh Epidemiology of Diabetes Complications Study, 658 patients with type 1 diabetes were evaluated [6]. During a median 20-year follow-up period, mortality was 6.2 (95% confidence interval (CI); 5.2–7.2) times higher than that in the age- and sex-matched general population, with standardized mortality ratios of 2.0 (95%

K. Muta · Y. Obata · T. Nishino (✉)
Department of Nephrology, Nagasaki University Hospital, Nagasaki, Japan
e-mail: tnishino@nagasaki-u.ac.jp

T. Wada et al. (eds.), *Diabetic Kidney Disease*,
https://doi.org/10.1007/978-981-15-9301-7_3

CI; 1.2–2.8) for normoalbuminuria, 6.4 (95% CI; 4.4–8.4) for microalbuminuria (20–200 μg/min), 12.5 (95% CI; 9.5–15.4) for overt nephropathy (>200 μg/min), and 29.8 (95% CI; 16.8–42.9) for ESRD (dialysis or renal transplantation) [6]. In the Third National Health and Nutrition Examination Survey (NHANES III) including 15,046 participants with type 2 diabetes, among individuals with both diabetes and kidney disease, the standardized 10-year cumulative mortality rate was 31.1% (95% CI; 24.7–37.5), representing an absolute risk difference consisting of people with no diabetes or kidney disease of 23.4% (95% CI; 14.7–29.6) after adjusting for age, sex, race, smoking, blood pressure, and cholesterol [7]. Among patients with diabetes and no kidney disease, no significant difference was observed in standardized mortality compared to the reference group consisting of people with no diabetes or kidney disease [7]. Thus, these studies showed that mortality is more strongly associated with the presence of kidney disease in patients with diabetes.

It has been recognized that albuminuria and reduced GFR are each associated with the development of CVD in patients with diabetes. The urinary albumin-to-creatinine ratio (UACR) levels increased the adjusted HR for cardiovascular events and all-cause mortality in a historical cohort study of 4328 Japanese participants with type 2 diabetes from ten centers [8]. Also in a meta-analysis of 31 cohort studies including diabetic patients, microalbuminuria (relative risk 1.76, 95% CI; 1.38–2.25) and macroalbuminuria (relative risk 2.96, 95% CI; 2.44–3.60) were significant risk factors of cardiovascular mortality compared to normoalbuminuria [9]. In a multicenter, large-scale cohort including 3002 Japanese patients with type 2 diabetes without macroalbuminuria, patients with an eGFR reduction without microalbuminuria had a twofold higher prevalence of CVD compared to patients without reduced eGFR and microalbuminuria (odds ratio 1.97) and similarly higher in those with microalbuminuria without reduced eGFR (odds ratio 1.85) [10]. In the Action in Diabetes and Vascular disease, the preterAx and diamicroN-MR Controlled Evaluation (ADVANCE) study, the effects of the UACR and eGFR on the risk for cardiovascular events in patients with type 2 diabetes were investigated [11]. During a median 4.3-year follow-up period, the multivariable-adjusted HR for cardiovascular events was 2.48 (95% CI; 1.74–3.52) for every tenfold increase in baseline UACR and 2.20 (95% CI; 1.09–4.43) for every half of baseline eGFR [11]. Therefore, it has been shown that albuminuria and eGFR are independently associated with the development of CVD in patients with diabetes.

3.2 Risk Factors and Mechanisms of CVD in DKD

The risk factors for the development of CVD in patients with diabetes and CKD have been variably discussed. In the cross-sectional study of 1041 dialysis patients compared to the general population from the NHANES III, derived from baseline data of the Choices for Healthy Outcomes in Caring for ESRD (CHOICE), the prevalent risk factors for atherosclerotic CVD are diabetes, hypertension, left ventricular hypertrophy by electrocardiogram, low physical activity, low HDL cholesterol, and hypertriglyceridemia [12]. These are so-called traditional risk factors for CVD. However, some traditional risk factors, for example, hypertension, obesity, and hyperlipidemia, were inversely associated with mortality in patients with CKD [13].

In addition, nontraditional risk factors contribute to CVD in patients with CKD. It was shown that hyperphosphatemia was associated with CVD among patients with and without CKD because vascular calcification could be caused due to hyperphosphatemia [14]. Higher plasma β_2 microglobulin levels, which were elevated in patients with kidney failure, were independently associated with overall and cardiovascular mortality and cardiovascular events [15]. The increase of other uremic toxins, like indoxyl sulfate and *p*-cresyl sulfate, was associated with coronary atherosclerosis in patients with type 2 diabetes [16]. As some other risk factors, increased artery stiffness was a predictor of CVD mortality and was associated with CKD in patients with type 2 diabetes [17, 18]. In another study of patients with diabetes, anemia was also shown as a risk factor for CVD in individuals with CKD, but not without CKD [19]. High C-reactive protein (CRP) and hypoalbuminemia, which are inflammation factors, were independently associated with all-cause mortality and high CRP, but not serum albumin, which was an independent predictor for CVD mortality in CKD [20]. Vascular endothelial dysfunction can be also defined a risk factor of CVD [21]. Diabetic patients could obtain a hypercoagulable state by the elevation of many clotting factors and the inhibition of the fibrinolytic system and can be associated with the risk of CVD [22]. Cardiac valve calcification is also a predictor of an increased all-cause mortality and cardiovascular death in dialysis patients [23]. It was reported that mitral annulus calcification was associated with chronic kidney disease in the Cardiovascular Health Study, a community-based cohort of adults $\geq$ age 65, a total of 3929 individuals [24]. Diabetes was associated with aortic valve calcification in 6780 people of Multi-Ethnic Study of Atherosclerosis [25]. Aortic and mitral valve calcification was highly prevalent among individuals with diabetic kidney disease (UACR > 30 μg/min) compared to nondiabetic controls in a cross-sectional, case-control study of 32 individuals with type 2 diabetes and diabetic kidney disease [26]. From the above studies, cardiac valve calcification can be an important factor of increased CVD risk in patients with diabetes and/or CKD. We show risk factors of CVD in DKD patients in Table 3.1.

The mechanisms of CVD development in patients with DKD have remained unknown. Oxidative stress could be an important factor. Increased glucose and free

Table 3.1 Risk factors of cardiovascular disease in diabetic kidney disease patients

Diabetes	Stiffness of artery
Hypertension	Anemia
Dyslipidemia	High C-reactive protein
Left ventricular hypertrophy	Hypoalbuminemia
Low physical activity	Vascular endothelial dysfunction
Hyperphosphatemia	Hypercoagulable state
Uremic toxins	Cardiac valve calcification

fatty acids in diabetes increase free radical generation (oxidative stress), and oxidative stress induces endothelial dysfunction and insulin resistance, which may lead to CVD [27]. Inflammation can also be a key role to CVD contribution. In diabetes, the release of cytokines may be greater by activating macrophage, and cytokines increase the synthesis of the platelet-activating factor and stimulate the expression of adhesion molecules, inducing atherosclerosis [28]. It has also been reported that immune complexes with modified lipoproteins induce a large amount of cytokines and stimulate the expression of matrix metalloproteinase-1 and are associated with the development of CVD in diabetes [28]. Uremia can also increase oxidative stress and inflammation and contribute to an increased risk of CVD [29]. Uremic solutes, such as β_2 microglobulins, homocysteine, and cysteine, may become substrates for oxidative injury [29]. As the mechanism for the hypercoagulable state that contributes to CVD in diabetes, it was reported that increases in factor VII activity are related to increases in postprandial hyperlipidemia, and plasminogen activator inhibitor-1 overexpression may occur due to the effects of insulin and proinsulin [28].

Vascular calcification is an important pathological condition that contributes to the risk of CVD [30]. As the process to contribute to CVD in patients with CKD, endogenous inhibitors of calcification may be lacking in the uremic state [30]. Fibroblast growth factor 23 (FGF23), a phosphaturic hormone, might play a key role to contribute to the development of CVD in patients with CKD, because FGF23 enhances phosphate-induced vascular calcification by promoting osteoblastic differentiation [31]. In addition, uremia may impair cardiovascular repair mechanisms in patients with advanced renal failure [32].

3.3 Manifestation of CVD in DKD

CVD generally includes underlying diseases such as coronary artery disease and myocardial infarction, congestive heart failure, stroke, atrial fibrillation, peripheral arterial disease, and sudden cardiac death. The association between these diseases, diabetes and CKD, was verified. For example, incidence of myocardial infarction, stroke, and cardiovascular death was 25.0%, and incidence of chronic heart failure hospitalization was 8.5% among individuals with a history of diabetes mellitus and microalbuminuria in the Heart Outcomes Prevention Evaluation Study, a cohort study of participants aged 55 years or more with a history of CVD (n = 5545) or diabetes mellitus and at least one cardiovascular risk factor (n = 3498) with a median 4.5 years of follow-up [33]. Sudden cardiac death was the most common cause of death, accounting for 25% in 1255 patients with type 2 diabetes mellitus receiving maintenance hemodialysis who were randomly assigned to receive atorvastatin or placebo in a multicenter, randomized, double-blind, prospective study [34]. Diabetes was also one of the risk factors for cerebrovascular disease in dialysis patients [35]. Likewise, some cardiovascular complications can be developed in patients with diabetes and CKD.

3.4 Prevention and Management to Reduce CVD Risk

To prevent the development of CVD in patients with diabetes and CKD, multifactorial therapy is important to control the related factors, for example, hypertension, albuminuria, hyperglycemia, and dyslipidemia. We show management of CVD risk factors in DKD based on some guidelines in Table 3.2.

3.4.1 Management of Hyperglycemia

Hyperglycemia is the most important therapeutic target in patients with diabetes. In *Standards of Medical Care in Diabetes* by the American Diabetes Association, a glycosylated hemoglobin (HbA1c) of <7.0% is recommended to reduce the incidence of microvascular diseases [36]. Further, more stringent HbA1c targets (<6.5%) are considered in selected patients, if possible without significant hypoglycemia or other adverse effects of treatment [36]. Less stringent HbA1c goals (<8.0%) are appropriate for patients with a history of severe hypoglycemia, limited life expectancy, advanced complications, extensive comorbid conditions, and those where the goal is difficult to achieve despite diabetes self-management education,

Table 3.2 Management of CVD risk factors in DKD based on guidelines

Risk factor	Guideline	Management recommendation
Poor control of blood glucose	ADA [36]	• HbA1c <7.0% to reduce the incidence of microvascular diseases • More stringent HbA1c targets (<6.5%) in patients without significant hypoglycemia or other adverse effects of treatment • Less stringent HbA1c goals (<8.0%) for patients with a history of severe hypoglycemia, limited life expectancy, advanced complications, extensive comorbid conditions, and those in whom the goal is difficult to achieve
	AACE/ ACE [37]	HbA1C level ≤6.5% for most nonpregnant adults
Hypertension	KDGIO [38]	• Less than 140/90 mmHg in adults with diabetes and CKD without albuminuria • Less than 130/80 mmHg in those with albuminuria • Recommendation of the use of angiotensin receptor blocker and ACE inhibitor in adults with diabetes and CKD with albuminuria
	ADA [36]	• Less than 140/90 mmHg in patients with diabetes and hypertension • Lower blood pressure targets (130/80 mmHg) for individuals at high risk of cardiovascular disease • First-line recommendation of an ACE inhibitor or angiotensin receptor blocker, at the maximum tolerated dose in patients with diabetes and albuminuria

(continued)

Table 3.2 (continued)

Risk factor	Guideline	Management recommendation
Albuminuria	KDOQI [39]	• Recommendation of using an ACE inhibitor or an angiotensin receptor blocker in normotensive patients with diabetes and albuminuria levels >30 mg/g who are at high risk of DKD or its progression
Dyslipidemia	AACE/ACE [40]	• LDL cholesterol goal <130 mg/dL at lower risk, <100 mg/dL at moderate risk and high risk, <75 mg/dL at very high risk, and <55 mg/dL at extreme risk • Triglyceride goal <150 mg/dL and HDL cholesterol >40 mg/dL
	KDIGO [41] ACC/AHA [42]	No recommendation of specific serum LDL cholesterol level for lipid-lowering therapy with statin
Salt intake	WHO [43]	Reduce salt intake by 5 g/day to prevent CVD in adults and children
	ADA [36]	Sodium consumption to 2300 mg/day in patients with diabetes and hypertension
Protein intake	ADA [36]	Dietary protein at 0.8 g/kg body weight/day for people with diabetic kidney disease
Smoking	ADA [36]	Not to use cigarettes and other tobacco products or e-cigarettes
Alcohol	ADA [36]	No major detrimental effects of moderate alcohol consumption on long-term blood glucose control in people with diabetes

AACE/ACE American Association of Clinical Endocrinologists and American College of Endocrinology, *ACC/AHA* American College of Cardiology and American Heart Association, *ACE* angiotensin-converting enzyme, *ADA* American Diabetes Association, *CKD* chronic kidney disease, *CVD* cardiovascular disease, *DKD* diabetic kidney disease, *HbA1c* hemoglobin A1c, *HDL* high-density lipoprotein, *KDIGO* Kidney Disease: Improving Global Outcomes, *KDOQI* Kidney Disease Outcomes Quality Initiative, *LDL* low-density lipoprotein, *WHO* World Health Organization

appropriate glucose monitoring, and effective doses of multiple glucose-lowering agents including insulin [36]. However, the effect of glycemic control on the inhibition of CVD risk has not been clearly proven. In the Diabetes Control and Complications Trial, a multicenter, randomized clinical trial designed to compare intensive and conventional diabetes therapies, intensive therapy reduced the risk of macrovascular events by 41%, although not significantly, in patients with type 1 diabetes [44]. In the Steno-2 study, a randomized controlled trial that evaluated patients with type 2 diabetes and albuminuria, the effect of a targeted, intensified, multifactorial intervention with that of conventional treatment on risk factors of CVD was compared [45]. In the end of this study, intensive therapy significantly reduced HbA1c values compared to conventional therapy (HbA1c values in the end of study; intensive therapy 7.9%, conventional therapy 9.0%, $p < 0.001$) [45]. In addition, the risk of CVD development was significantly lower when patients underwent intensive therapy [45]. However, the rate that achieved an HbA1c of 6.5%, the goal of this study, was very low in the intensive therapy patients.

Therefore, we cannot conclude that the effect of glycemic control on the inhibition of CVD risk was shown [45].

Regarding the effect of glycemic control on the inhibition of CVD risk, the reduction in albuminuria by glycemic control may be associated. In a prospective observational study of 216 Japanese patients with type 2 diabetes and microalbuminuria, reductions in the urinary albumin excretion rate were frequent, with a 6-year cumulative incidence of 51% (95% CI; 42–60) for remission and 54% (95% CI; 45–63) for regression, whereas the frequency of progression to overt proteinuria was 28% (95% CI; 19–37) [46]. Lower tertiles for HbA1c (<6.95%) were independently associated with remission or regression of microalbuminuria in the pooled logistic regression analysis [46]. In another 2-year follow-up of this study, the cumulative incidence of CVD was significantly lower in the microalbuminuria remission group at least once during the follow-up period than in the non-remission group [47].

From the above observations, although the effect of glycemic control on the inhibition of CVD development has remained unknown, glycemic control can play a key contributing role to reduce CVD risk as a central factor for intensified, multifactorial therapy of diabetes and CKD and as a factor of remission of albuminuria.

3.4.2 New Glucose-Lowering Therapies and CVD

Recently numerous large randomized controlled cardiovascular outcome trials have been published in type 2 diabetes with CVD or at high risk of CVD using new glucose-lowering therapies such as sodium-glucose cotransporter 2 (SGLT2) inhibitors, glucagon-like peptidase 1 (GLP-1) receptor agonists, and dipeptidyl peptidase 4 inhibitors. Especially, the results from trials using SGLT2 inhibitors and GLP-1 receptor agonists have shown beneficial effects of these drugs to cardiovascular outcome in patients with type 2 diabetes and CKD.

First, as a famous SGLT2 inhibitor trial, Empagliflozin Cardiovascular Outcome Event Trial in Type 2 Diabetes Mellitus Patients (EMPA-REG OUTCOME) was a randomized, double-blind, placebo-controlled trial to assess the effect of empagliflozin versus placebo on cardiovascular events in adults with type 2 diabetes at high cardiovascular risk against a background of standard care [48]. In a post hoc analysis of this trial, empagliflozin reduced the risk of cardiovascular death by 29% in patients with prevalent kidney disease at baseline (defined as eGFR <60 mL/min/1.73 m^2 and/or urine albumin-creatinine ratio > 300 mg/g) compared with placebo (HR, 0.71; 95% CI, 0.52–0.98) and the risk of hospitalization for heart failure by 39% (HR, 0.61; 95% CI, 0.42–0.87) [49]. Even in a post hoc analysis of data from CANagliflozin cardioVascular Assessment Study (CANVAS) that is a double-blind comparison of the effects of canagliflozin versus placebo, the effect of canagliflozin on the composite of cardiovascular death, nonfatal myocardial infarction, or nonfatal stroke, with other cardiovascular, renal, and safety outcomes was similar in people with CKD (eGFR < 60 mL/min/1.73 m^2) (HR, 0.70; 95% CI, 0.55–0.90) and those with preserved kidney function (>60 mL/min/1.73 m^2) (HR, 0.92; 95% CI, 0.79–1.07; p heterogeneity = 0.08) [50]. Furthermore, Canagliflozin and Renal Events in Diabetes with Established Nephropathy Clinical Evaluation (CREDENCE) trial was a double-blind, randomized trial in patients with type 2 diabetes and albuminuric CKD (eGFR of 30 to <90 mL/min/1.73 m^2 and albuminuria (>300–5000 mg/gCr) and treated with renin-angiotensin system blockade) to receive canagliflozin or placebo [51]. The canagliflozin group had a lower risk of cardiovascular death, myocardial infarction, or stroke (HR, 0.80; 95% CI, 0.67–0.95; $p = 0.01$) and hospitalization for heart failure (HR, 0.61; 95% CI, 0.47–0.80; $p < 0.001$) compared to those of placebo group [51]. The results of these three trials showed that SGLT2 inhibitors could be beneficial in patients with diabetes and CKD to inhibit CVD.

Next, as for GLP-1 receptor agonist, Liraglutide Effect and Action in Diabetes: Evaluation of CV Outcome Results (LEADER) trial was a multicenter, double-blind, placebo-controlled trial that patients were randomized (1:1) to liraglutide or placebo, both in addition to standard of care [52]. In a post hoc analysis of this trial, these analyses assessed outcomes stratified by baseline eGFR (eGFR; <60 versus ≥60 mL/min/1.73 m^2) and baseline albuminuria [53]. In patients with eGFR <60 mL/min/1.73 m^2, risk reduction for the primary composite cardiovascular outcome with liraglutide was greater (HR, 0.69; 95% CI, 0.57–0.85) versus those with eGFR ≥ 60 mL/min/1.73 m^2 (HR, 0.94; 95% CI, 0.83–1.07; interaction $p = 0.01$). Risk reduction for the primary composite cardiovascular outcome was not different for those with versus without baseline albuminuria (HR, 0.83; 95% CI, 0.71–0.97; and HR, 0.92; 95% CI, 0.79–1.07, respectively; interaction $p = 0.36$) [53].

These analyses showed that SGLT2 inhibitors and GLP-1 agonists in patients with type 2 diabetes and CKD might lead to a reduction of CV outcomes.

3.4.3 Management of Hypertension

In general, the risk of CVD is reduced by the treatment for hypertension. In a prospective observational study for patients with type 2 diabetes, each 10 mmHg decrease in mean systolic blood pressure was associated with the reduction of CVD and mortality [54]. On the other hand, in the Irbesartan Diabetic Nephropathy Trial (IDNT), a randomized, double-blind, placebo-controlled trial using data from 1590 hypertensive patients with type 2 diabetes, the relative risk of all-cause mortality was the lowest in patients with an average follow-up blood pressure of 121–130 mmHg [55]. In IDNT, patients with the lowest follow-up SBP (<120 mmHg) had sharply higher mortality [55]. In the Action to Control Cardiovascular Risk in Diabetes, a randomized trial including 4733 participants with type 2 diabetes, the rate of composite outcomes of fatal and nonfatal major cardiovascular events did not decrease in the intensive therapy targeting a systolic pressure of less than 120 mmHg, compared to standard therapy targeting a systolic pressure of less than 140 mmHg [56]. However, the annual stroke rate significantly decreased in intensive therapy compared to standard therapy [56]. In regard to strokes, intensive blood pressure control (≤130 mmHg) was associated with a greater reduction in strokes from a meta-regression analysis [30].

Based on the data from studies, including the ones mentioned above, Kidney Disease: Improving Global Outcomes Blood Pressure (KDIGO-BP) guideline recommends a blood pressure of less than 140/90 mmHg in adults with diabetes and CKD without albuminuria [38].

3.4.4 Management of Albuminuria

As another role of blood pressure control to prohibit CVD risk, lowering blood pressure reduces the rate of urinary albumin excretion [38]. Albuminuria is associated with the development of CVD in patients with diabetes [8–11].

In the KDIGO-BP guideline, the goal is less than 130/80 mmHg in adults with diabetes and CKD with albuminuria [38]. The use of angiotensin receptor blockers and angiotensin-converting enzyme inhibitors is recommended to control hypertension and albuminuria in those people [38].

3.4.5 Management of Dyslipidemia

Dyslipidemia is an important factor for CVD risk in the general population and is common in patients with diabetes and CKD. A condition of diabetes-related dyslipidemia includes hypertriglyceridemia, low high-density lipoprotein (HDL) levels, and increases in small and dense low-density lipoprotein (LDL) particles [57]. These lipid abnormalities can induce the development of CVD [57]. Related to CKD, from the data in the population-based Atherosclerosis Risk in Communities Study, a population-based prospective cohort study of 807 participants with CKD, higher levels of total cholesterol and triglycerides were associated with an increased coronary heart disease risk [58]. In an observational study with 45,390 hemodialysis patients, incident myocardial infarction was positively associated with non-HDL cholesterol and inversely with HDL cholesterol [59].

Lowering cholesterol using statin treatment is useful to inhibit CVD risk. In the Collaborative Atorvastatin Diabetes Study, a randomized placebo-controlled trial of 2838 patients with type 2 diabetes, it was showed that lowering LDL cholesterol reduced cardiovascular events in those with and without a moderately decreased eGFR [60]. The Study of Heart and Renal Protection trial, a randomized double-blind trial including 9270 patients with CKD (3023 on dialysis and 6247 not on dialysis), with allocation to receive simvastatin and ezetimibe, produced a 17% proportion reduction in major atherosclerotic events during a median follow-up of 4.9 years (526 [11.3%] simvastatin plus ezetimibe versus 619 [13.4%] placebo; rate ratio 0.83, 95% CI; 0.74–0.94; log-rank $p = 0.0021$) [61]. However, there was no significant reduction in major atherosclerotic events in patients on dialysis [61].

Similarly, the administration of statins did not significantly reduce the risk of CVD in patients on dialysis in two other randomized controlled trials [34, 62]. Conversely, some randomized controlled trials showed that CVD risk significantly decreased using statin treatment in patients with CKD stage G3 (eGFR 30–60 mL/min/1.73 m^2) [63–65]. Therefore, it is better that treatment with statin is initiated in patients with predialysis CKD to inhibit the risk of CVD.

The treatment goal for dyslipidemia in patients at risk for atherosclerotic CVD is personalized according to levels of risk according to the American Association of Clinical Endocrinologists and American College of Endocrinology Management of Dyslipidemia and Prevention of Cardiovascular Disease Writing Committee [40]. An LDL cholesterol goal is recommended at <130 mg/dL for those with a lower risk, <100 mg/dL for those with a moderate or high risk, <75 mg/dL for those with a very high risk, and <55 mg/dL for extreme risk patients [40]. A triglyceride goal of <150 mg/dL and HDL cholesterol goal of >40 mg/dL are recommended [40]. On the other hand, specific serum LDL cholesterol levels have not been recommended for lipid-lowering therapies with statin in guidelines like the KDIGO 2013 Clinical Practice Guidelines and American College of Cardiology and American Heart Association Guideline [41, 42]. This is because the association with LDL cholesterol and coronary risk was weaker and potentially misleading among patients with lower levels of kidney function [41]. Statin treatment should be considered in most patients with diabetes and CKD to prevent or inhibit CVD development.

3.4.6 Multifactorial Therapy

To reduce the risk of CVD, an intensified, multifactorial intervention that targets hyperglycemia, hypertension, and dyslipidemia is recommended in patients with diabetes and CKD, as shown in the above Steno-2 study [45].

3.4.7 Lifestyle

To prevent and inhibit CVD risk, lifestyle changes are recommended in patients with diabetes and CKD. Decreasing salt intake reduces the long-term risk of CVD [43]. In a meta-analysis of 19 prospective cohorts with 177,025 participants, a higher salt intake was associated with an increased risk of stroke and CVD [66]. The World Health Organization (WHO) recommends to reduce salt intake by 5 g/day to prevent CVD in adults and children [43]. However, a multicenter study with 2807 patients with type 1 diabetes showed that salt intake estimated by urinary sodium excretion was nonlinearly associated with all-cause mortality, that is, both individuals with the highest and lowest daily urinary sodium excretion had reduced survival [67]. Therefore, not only a higher salt intake but also an excessive lower salt intake should be avoided to reduce mortality and development of CVD.

For people with DKD, dietary protein is recommended to be maintained at 0.8 g/kg body weight/day [36]. Reducing the amount of dietary protein below the recommended daily allowance is not recommended because it does not alter cardiovascular risk measures [36].

Smoking is related to the risk of CVD. In a meta-analysis of 34 cohorts involving 16,492 participants with diabetes and 188,897 participants without diabetes, smoking cessation reduced 19% of the CV risk [68]. Therefore, smoking cessation is recommended to prevent CVD risk.

Excess alcohol intake is associated with liver disease, cancer, suicide, and so on [69]. A J-shaped relationship was shown between alcohol consumption and CV mortality, which was maximal in the range of 5–10 g/day and was significant up to approximately 26 g/day, in a meta-analysis including 16,351 patients with a history of CVD [70]. Whereas, in an Australian population-representative study of 6259 adults ≥25 years of age, alcohol intake of ≥30 g/day was associated with an increased risk of albuminuria after adjustment for age, sex, and baseline kidney function (odds ratio 1.59, 95% CI; 1.07–2.36), but alcohol intake of ≥30 g/day reduced risk of eGFR <60 (odds ratio 0.59, 95% CI; 0.37–0.95), compared with consumption of <10 g/day [71]. In another cohort study including 4,343 participants aged ≥65 from US communities, there was no association between alcohol use and kidney function decline [72]. Therefore, little or moderate alcohol intake may affect kidney function preservation and reduce the development of CVD.

3.4.8 *Management of CVD*

Cardiovascular complications are widely observed in patients with CKD. A report on conference proceedings and recommendations about CVD in CKD was published from KDIGO in 2011 [73]. Epidemiology, pathology, diagnosis, prevention, and treatment of CVD, including coronary artery disease and myocardial infarction, congestive heart failure, cerebrovascular disease, atrial fibrillation, peripheral arterial disease, and sudden cardiac death, were described in patients with CKD in the report [73]. Optimized strategies of prevention, diagnosis, and management of CVD should be determined by more future trials.

3.5 Conclusion

The presence of DKD is strongly associated with the development of CVD. However, the mechanism of why CVD risk is elevated in patients with diabetes and CKD should be further investigated, and the management of patients with diabetes and CKD should be continued more carefully and widely to prevent and inhibit the development of CVD.

References

1. Grundy SM, Benjamin IJ, Burke GL, Chait A, Eckel RH, Howard BV, et al. Diabetes and cardiovascular disease: a statement for healthcare professionals from the American Heart Association. Circulation. 1999;100(10):1134–46.
2. Rao Kondapally Seshasai S, Kaptoge S, Thompson A, Di Angelantonio E, Gao P, Sarwar N, et al. Diabetes mellitus, fasting glucose, and risk of cause-specific death. N Engl J Med. 2011;364(9):829–41.
3. Sarnak MJ, Levey AS, Schoolwerth AC, Coresh J, Culleton B, Hamm LL, et al. Kidney disease as a risk factor for development of cardiovascular disease: a statement from the American Heart Association Councils on Kidney in Cardiovascular Disease, High Blood Pressure Research, Clinical Cardiology, and Epidemiology and Prevention. Circulation. 2003;108(17):2154–69.
4. Eriksen BO, Ingebretsen OC. The progression of chronic kidney disease: a 10-year population-based study of the effects of gender and age. Kidney Int. 2006;69(2):375–82.
5. Groop PH, Thomas MC, Moran JL, Waden J, Thorn LM, Makinen VP, et al. The presence and severity of chronic kidney disease predicts all-cause mortality in type 1 diabetes. Diabetes. 2009;58(7):1651–8.
6. Orchard TJ, Secrest AM, Miller RG, Costacou T. In the absence of renal disease, 20 year mortality risk in type 1 diabetes is comparable to that of the general population: a report from the Pittsburgh Epidemiology of Diabetes Complications Study. Diabetologia. 2010;53(11):2312–9.
7. Afkarian M, Sachs MC, Kestenbaum B, Hirsch IB, Tuttle KR, Himmelfarb J, et al. Kidney disease and increased mortality risk in type 2 diabetes. J Am Soc Nephrol. 2013;24(2):302–8.
8. Wada T, Haneda M, Furuichi K, Babazono T, Yokoyama H, Iseki K, et al. Clinical impact of albuminuria and glomerular filtration rate on renal and cardiovascular events, and all-cause mortality in Japanese patients with type 2 diabetes. Clin Exp Nephrol. 2014;18(4):613–20.
9. Toyama T, Furuichi K, Ninomiya T, Shimizu M, Hara A, Iwata Y, et al. The impacts of albuminuria and low eGFR on the risk of cardiovascular death, all-cause mortality, and renal events in diabetic patients: meta-analysis. PLoS One. 2013;8(8):e71810.
10. Yokoyama H, Oishi M, Kawai K, Sone H. Reduced GFR and microalbuminuria are independently associated with prevalent cardiovascular disease in Type 2 diabetes: JDDM study 16. Diabet Med. 2008;25(12):1426–32.
11. Ninomiya T, Perkovic V, de Galan BE, Zoungas S, Pillai A, Jardine M, et al. Albuminuria and kidney function independently predict cardiovascular and renal outcomes in diabetes. J Am Soc Nephrol. 2009;20(8):1813–21.
12. Longenecker JC, Coresh J, Powe NR, Levey AS, Fink NE, Martin A, et al. Traditional cardiovascular disease risk factors in dialysis patients compared with the general population: the CHOICE Study. J Am Soc Nephrol. 2002;13(7):1918–27.
13. Kovesdy CP, Anderson JE. Reverse epidemiology in patients with chronic kidney disease who are not yet on dialysis. Semin Dial. 2007;20(6):566–9.
14. Kendrick J, Kestenbaum B, Chonchol M. Phosphate and cardiovascular disease. Adv Chronic Kidney Dis. 2011;18(2):113–9.
15. Liabeuf S, Lenglet A, Desjardins L, Neirynck N, Glorieux G, Lemke HD, et al. Plasma beta-2 microglobulin is associated with cardiovascular disease in uremic patients. Kidney Int. 2012;82(12):1297–303.
16. Chiu CA, Lu LF, Yu TH, Hung WC, Chung FM, Tsai IT, et al. Increased levels of total P-Cresylsulphate and indoxyl sulphate are associated with coronary artery disease in patients with diabetic nephropathy. Rev Diabet Stud. 2010;7(4):275–84.
17. Shoji T, Emoto M, Shinohara K, Kakiya R, Tsujimoto Y, Kishimoto H, et al. Diabetes mellitus, aortic stiffness, and cardiovascular mortality in end-stage renal disease. J Am Soc Nephrol. 2001;12(10):2117–24.
18. Kimoto E, Shoji T, Shinohara K, Hatsuda S, Mori K, Fukumoto S, et al. Regional arterial stiffness in patients with type 2 diabetes and chronic kidney disease. J Am Soc Nephrol. 2006;17(8):2245–52.

19. Vlagopoulos PT, Tighiouart H, Weiner DE, Griffith J, Pettitt D, Salem DN, et al. Anemia as a risk factor for cardiovascular disease and all-cause mortality in diabetes: the impact of chronic kidney disease. J Am Soc Nephrol. 2005;16(11):3403–10.
20. Menon V, Greene T, Wang X, Pereira AA, Marcovina SM, Beck GJ, et al. C-reactive protein and albumin as predictors of all-cause and cardiovascular mortality in chronic kidney disease. Kidney Int. 2005;68(2):766–72.
21. Stehouwer CD, Smulders YM. Microalbuminuria and risk for cardiovascular disease: analysis of potential mechanisms. J Am Soc Nephrol. 2006;17(8):2106–11.
22. Carr ME. Diabetes mellitus: a hypercoagulable state. J Diabetes Complications. 2001;15(1):44–54.
23. Wang AY, Wang M, Woo J, Lam CW, Li PK, Lui SF, et al. Cardiac valve calcification as an important predictor for all-cause mortality and cardiovascular mortality in long-term peritoneal dialysis patients: a prospective study. J Am Soc Nephrol. 2003;14(1):159–68.
24. Asselbergs FW, Mozaffarian D, Katz R, Kestenbaum B, Fried LF, Gottdiener JS, et al. Association of renal function with cardiac calcifications in older adults: the cardiovascular health study. Nephrol Dial Transplant. 2009;24(3):834–40.
25. Katz R, Wong ND, Kronmal R, Takasu J, Shavelle DM, Probstfield JL, et al. Features of the metabolic syndrome and diabetes mellitus as predictors of aortic valve calcification in the Multi-Ethnic Study of Atherosclerosis. Circulation. 2006;113(17):2113–9.
26. Merjanian R, Budoff M, Adler S, Berman N, Mehrotra R. Coronary artery, aortic wall, and valvular calcification in nondialyzed individuals with type 2 diabetes and renal disease. Kidney Int. 2003;64(1):263–71.
27. Ceriello A, Motz E. Is oxidative stress the pathogenic mechanism underlying insulin resistance, diabetes, and cardiovascular disease? The common soil hypothesis revisited. Arterioscler Thromb Vasc Biol. 2004;24(5):816–23.
28. Eckel RH, Wassef M, Chait A, Sobel B, Barrett E, King G, et al. Prevention conference VI: diabetes and cardiovascular disease: writing group II: pathogenesis of atherosclerosis in diabetes. Circulation. 2002;105(18):e138–43.
29. Himmelfarb J, Stenvinkel P, Ikizler TA, Hakim RM. The elephant in uremia: oxidant stress as a unifying concept of cardiovascular disease in uremia. Kidney Int. 2002;62(5):1524–38.
30. Bangalore S, Kumar S, Lobach I, Messerli FH. Blood pressure targets in subjects with type 2 diabetes mellitus/impaired fasting glucose: observations from traditional and bayesian random-effects meta-analyses of randomized trials. Circulation. 2011;123(24):2799–810.
31. Jimbo R, Shimosawa T. Cardiovascular risk factors and chronic kidney disease-FGF23: a key molecule in the cardiovascular disease. Int J Hypertens. 2014;2014:381082.
32. de Groot K, Bahlmann FH, Sowa J, Koenig J, Menne J, Haller H, et al. Uremia causes endothelial progenitor cell deficiency. Kidney Int. 2004;66(2):641–6.
33. Gerstein HC, Mann JF, Yi Q, Zinman B, Dinneen SF, Hoogwerf B, et al. Albuminuria and risk of cardiovascular events, death, and heart failure in diabetic and nondiabetic individuals. JAMA. 2001;286(4):421–6.
34. Wanner C, Krane V, Marz W, Olschewski M, Mann JF, Ruf G, et al. Atorvastatin in patients with type 2 diabetes mellitus undergoing hemodialysis. N Engl J Med. 2005;353(3):238–48.
35. Sozio SM, Armstrong PA, Coresh J, Jaar BG, Fink NE, Plantinga LC, et al. Cerebrovascular disease incidence, characteristics, and outcomes in patients initiating dialysis: the choices for healthy outcomes in caring for ESRD (CHOICE) study. Am J Kidney Dis. 2009;54(3):468–77.
36. American Diabetes Association. Standards of medical care in diabetes-2020. Diabetes Care. 2020;43(Suppl 1):S1–S212.
37. Handelsman Y, Bloomgarden ZT, Grunberger G, Umpierrez G, Zimmerman RS, Bailey TS, et al. American association of clinical endocrinologists and American college of endocrinology—clinical practice guidelines for developing a diabetes mellitus comprehensive care plan—2015. Endocr Pract. 2015;21(Suppl 1):1–87.

38. Kidney Disease: Improving Global Outcomes (KDIGO) Blood Pressure Work Group. KDIGO clinical practice guideline for the management of blood pressure in chronic kidney disease. Kidney Int Suppl. 2012;2:337–414.
39. National Kidney Foundation. KDOQI Clinical Practice Guideline for Diabetes and CKD: 2012 Update. Am J Kidney Dis. 2012;60(5):850–86.
40. Jellinger PS, Handelsman Y, Rosenblit PD, Bloomgarden ZT, Fonseca VA, Garber AJ, et al. American Association of Clinical Endocrinologists and American College of Endocrinology guidelines for management of dyslipidemia and prevention of cardiovascular disease. Endocr Pract. 2017;23(Suppl 2):1–87.
41. Tonelli M, Wanner C. Lipid management in chronic kidney disease: synopsis of the Kidney Disease: Improving Global Outcomes 2013 clinical practice guideline. Ann Intern Med. 2014;160(3):182.
42. Grundy SM, Stone NJ, Bailey AL, Beam C, Birtcher KK, Blumenthal RS, et al. 2018 AHA/ACC/AACVPR/AAPA/ABC/ACPM/ADA/AGS/APhA/ASPC/NLA/PCNA guideline on the management of blood cholesterol: executive summary: a report of the American College of Cardiology/American Heart Association Task Force on Clinical Practice Guidelines. Circulation. 2019;139(25):e1046–e81.
43. WHO. Creating an enabling environment for population–based salt reduction strategies. 2010. p. 4–34.
44. Nathan DM, Genuth S, Lachin J, Cleary P, Crofford O, Davis M, et al. The effect of intensive treatment of diabetes on the development and progression of long-term complications in insulin-dependent diabetes mellitus. N Engl J Med. 1993;329(14):977–86.
45. Gaede P, Vedel P, Larsen N, Jensen GV, Parving HH, Pedersen O. Multifactorial intervention and cardiovascular disease in patients with type 2 diabetes. N Engl J Med. 2003;348(5):383–93.
46. Araki S, Haneda M, Sugimoto T, Isono M, Isshiki K, Kashiwagi A, et al. Factors associated with frequent remission of microalbuminuria in patients with type 2 diabetes. Diabetes. 2005;54(10):2983–7.
47. Araki S, Haneda M, Koya D, Hidaka H, Sugimoto T, Isono M, et al. Reduction in microalbuminuria as an integrated indicator for renal and cardiovascular risk reduction in patients with type 2 diabetes. Diabetes. 2007;56(6):1727–30.
48. Zinman B, Wanner C, Lachin JM, Fitchett D, Bluhmki E, Hantel S, et al. Empagliflozin, cardiovascular outcomes, and mortality in type 2 diabetes. N Engl J Med. 2015;373(22):2117–28.
49. Wanner C, Lachin JM, Inzucchi SE, Fitchett D, Mattheus M, George J, et al. Empagliflozin and clinical outcomes in patients with type 2 diabetes mellitus, established cardiovascular disease, and chronic kidney disease. Circulation. 2018;137(2):119–29.
50. Neuen BL, Ohkuma T, Neal B, Matthews DR, de Zeeuw D, Mahaffey KW, et al. Cardiovascular and renal outcomes with canagliflozin according to baseline kidney function. Circulation. 2018;138(15):1537–50.
51. Perkovic V, Jardine MJ, Neal B, Bompoint S, Heerspink HJL, Charytan DM, et al. Canagliflozin and renal outcomes in type 2 diabetes and nephropathy. N Engl J Med. 2019;380(24):2295–306.
52. Marso SP, Daniels GH, Brown-Frandsen K, Kristensen P, Mann JF, Nauck MA, et al. Liraglutide and cardiovascular outcomes in type 2 diabetes. N Engl J Med. 2016;375(4):311–22.
53. Mann JFE, Fonseca V, Mosenzon O, Raz I, Goldman B, Idorn T, et al. Effects of liraglutide versus placebo on cardiovascular events in patients with type 2 diabetes mellitus and chronic kidney disease. Circulation. 2018;138(25):2908–18.
54. Adler AI, Stratton IM, Neil HA, Yudkin JS, Matthews DR, Cull CA, et al. Association of systolic blood pressure with macrovascular and microvascular complications of type 2 diabetes (UKPDS 36): prospective observational study. BMJ. 2000;321(7258):412–9.
55. Pohl MA, Blumenthal S, Cordonnier DJ, De Alvaro F, Deferrari G, Eisner G, et al. Independent and additive impact of blood pressure control and angiotensin II receptor blockade on renal outcomes in the irbesartan diabetic nephropathy trial: clinical implications and limitations. J Am Soc Nephrol. 2005;16(10):3027–37.

56. Cushman WC, Evans GW, Byington RP, Goff DC Jr, Grimm RH Jr, Cutler JA, et al. Effects of intensive blood-pressure control in type 2 diabetes mellitus. N Engl J Med. 2010;362(17):1575–85.
57. Chen SC, Tseng CH. Dyslipidemia, kidney disease, and cardiovascular disease in diabetic patients. Rev Diabet Stud. 2013;10(2–3):88–100.
58. Muntner P, He J, Astor BC, Folsom AR, Coresh J. Traditional and nontraditional risk factors predict coronary heart disease in chronic kidney disease: results from the atherosclerosis risk in communities study. J Am Soc Nephrol. 2005;16(2):529–38.
59. Shoji T, Masakane I, Watanabe Y, Iseki K, Tsubakihara Y. Elevated non-high-density lipoprotein cholesterol (non-HDL-C) predicts atherosclerotic cardiovascular events in hemodialysis patients. Clin J Am Soc Nephrol. 2011;6(5):1112–20.
60. Colhoun HM, Betteridge DJ, Durrington PN, Hitman GA, Neil HA, Livingstone SJ, et al. Effects of atorvastatin on kidney outcomes and cardiovascular disease in patients with diabetes: an analysis from the Collaborative Atorvastatin Diabetes Study (CARDS). Am J Kidney Dis. 2009;54(5):810–9.
61. Baigent C, Landray MJ, Reith C, Emberson J, Wheeler DC, Tomson C, et al. The effects of lowering LDL cholesterol with simvastatin plus ezetimibe in patients with chronic kidney disease (Study of Heart and Renal Protection): a randomised placebo-controlled trial. Lancet. 2011;377(9784):2181–92.
62. Fellstrom BC, Jardine AG, Schmieder RE, Holdaas H, Bannister K, Beutler J, et al. Rosuvastatin and cardiovascular events in patients undergoing hemodialysis. N Engl J Med. 2009;360(14):1395–407.
63. Shepherd J, Kastelein JJ, Bittner V, Deedwania P, Breazna A, Dobson S, et al. Intensive lipid lowering with atorvastatin in patients with coronary heart disease and chronic kidney disease: the TNT (Treating to New Targets) study. J Am Coll Cardiol. 2008;51(15):1448–54.
64. Koren MJ, Davidson MH, Wilson DJ, Fayyad RS, Zuckerman A, Reed DP. Focused atorvastatin therapy in managed-care patients with coronary heart disease and CKD. Am J Kidney Dis. 2009;53(5):741–50.
65. Nakamura H, Mizuno K, Ohashi Y, Yoshida T, Hirao K, Uchida Y. Pravastatin and cardiovascular risk in moderate chronic kidney disease. Atherosclerosis. 2009;206(2):512–7.
66. Strazzullo P, D'Elia L, Kandala NB, Cappuccio FP. Salt intake, stroke, and cardiovascular disease: meta-analysis of prospective studies. BMJ. 2009;339:b4567.
67. Thomas MC, Moran J, Forsblom C, Harjutsalo V, Thorn L, Ahola A, et al. The association between dietary sodium intake, ESRD, and all-cause mortality in patients with type 1 diabetes. Diabetes Care. 2011;34(4):861–6.
68. Kengne AP, Nakamura K, Barzi F, Lam TH, Huxley R, Gu D, et al. Smoking, diabetes and cardiovascular diseases in men in the Asia Pacific region. J Diabetes. 2009;1(3):173–81.
69. Thun MJ, Peto R, Lopez AD, Monaco JH, Henley SJ, Heath CW Jr, et al. Alcohol consumption and mortality among middle-aged and elderly U.S. adults. N Engl J Med. 1997;337(24):1705–14.
70. Costanzo S, Di Castelnuovo A, Donati MB, Iacoviello L, de Gaetano G. Alcohol consumption and mortality in patients with cardiovascular disease: a meta-analysis. J Am Coll Cardiol. 2010;55(13):1339–47.
71. White SL, Polkinghorne KR, Cass A, Shaw JE, Atkins RC, Chadban SJ. Alcohol consumption and 5-year onset of chronic kidney disease: the AusDiab study. Nephrol Dial Transplant. 2009;24(8):2464–72.
72. Menon V, Katz R, Mukamal K, Kestenbaum B, de Boer IH, Siscovick DS, et al. Alcohol consumption and kidney function decline in the elderly: alcohol and kidney disease. Nephrol Dial Transplant. 2010;25(10):3301–7.
73. Herzog CA, Asinger RW, Berger AK, Charytan DM, Diez J, Hart RG, et al. Cardiovascular disease in chronic kidney disease. A clinical update from Kidney Disease: Improving Global Outcomes (KDIGO). Kidney Int. 2011;80(6):572–86.

Chapter 4
Possible Biomarkers for Diabetic Kidney Disease

Yukio Yuzawa and Daijo Inaguma

4.1 Introduction

The prevalence of diabetes is increasing worldwide and is the highest in the Western Pacific region, which includes Japan. The number of patients who require dialysis because of diabetic kidney disease (DKD) continues to increase. This warrants efforts to prevent the progression of DKD. Under these circumstances, there is an urgent need for the development of new DKD biomarkers, in addition to those currently available, for use in all phases of the disease, from early diagnosis and specific detection to prognostic prediction and assessment of treatment response.

Here, we describe biomarkers established using previously reported analytical methods and report on exploratory biomarkers and omics analyses for the development of novel biomarkers.

4.2 Biomarkers Currently Established Through the Use of Previously Reported Analytical Methods

Multiple biomarkers for DKD, including urine and serum biomarkers, have been described and validated [1] (Table 4.1).

Y. Yuzawa (✉) · D. Inaguma
Department of Nephrology, Fujita Health University School of Medicine, Toyoake, Aichi, Japan
e-mail: yukio-y@fujita-hu.ac.jp

T. Wada et al. (eds.), *Diabetic Kidney Disease*,
https://doi.org/10.1007/978-981-15-9301-7_4

Table 4.1 Characteristics of classical markers of DKD onset and progression

Marker		Sample	Characteristics
Glomerular injury markers			
Albumin		Urine	• Urinary albumin levels during the microalbuminuria stage are used to predict end-stage renal failure. Since there are wide variations in the data, there is low specificity for DKD ΔAER ≠ ΔGFR during the spontaneous regression and microalbuminuria stages
Type IV collagen		Urine	• Observed from the early stages of DKD. Consistent with tissue changes
Ceruloplasmin		Urine	• Urinary excretion increases prior to the appearance of albuminuria
GFR			• Best indicator of kidney function. There is currently no accurate method of estimating GFR levels that are within high normal range
Tubular injury markers			
NGAL		Urine	• Increased urinary excretion observed before the appearance of albuminuria
α1-MG		Urine	• Relatively inexpensive to measure
KIM-1		Urine	• Increased urinary excretion, even in cases of glomerular hyperfiltration, which is seen in early DKD
L-FABP		Urine	• Testing is covered by insurance, which has allowed its general use in clinical settings. Increased urinary excretion is observed in diabetes patients with normal urinary albumin levels
Angiotensinogen		Urine	• Increased urinary excretion is observed in diabetes patients with normal urinary albumin levels
Cystatin C		Urine	• Used in clinical settings as a marker for early kidney dysfunction as it is unaffected by muscle mass, age, or sex
NAG		Urine	• Commonly used in clinical settings to differentiate nephropathies
Inflammatory markers			
Inflammatory cytokines	IL-6	Blood/Urine	• Increased serum levels and urinary excretion levels prior to DKD onset or during early DKD
	IL-8	Blood/Urine	
	IL-18	Blood/Urine	
	IP-10	Blood/Urine	
	TNF-α	Blood/Urine	
	TNF-α receptor	Blood	

Table 4.1 (continued)

Marker	Sample		Characteristics
Growth factors	TGF-β	Urine	• Therapy leads to decreased urinary excretion
	CTGF	Blood/ Urine	• Related to urinary excretion of albumin and GFR. Related to end-stage renal failure and mortality
Adhesive factors	ICAM-1	Blood	• Related to albuminuria or microalbuminuria onset
	VCAM-1	Blood	
Fetuin-A		Blood/ Urine	• Related to albuminuria and decreased GFR
Soluble CD40 ligands		Blood/ Urine	• Elevated levels before sDKD onset
Human α1 acidic glycoprotein		Urine	• Increased urinary excretion during normal urinary albumin stage in diabetes patients
Oxidative stress markers			
8-OHdG		Urine	• Related to DKD progression
Pentosidine		Blood	• Related to microvascular lesions
Uric acid		Blood	• Can be a therapeutic target. Interventional study of kidney disease outcomes according to uric acid levels is necessary

4.2.1 Urine Biomarkers

4.2.1.1 Urine Albumin

In early DKD, glomerular endothelial cell proliferation is promoted by vascular endothelial growth factor (VEGF)-A. This results in capillary expansion and leads to glomerular hypertrophy [2]. The onset of glomerular epithelial cell damage eventually progresses to glomerulosclerosis. Similarly, hyperglycemia, advanced glycation end products, hypoxia, inflammation, and oxidative stress have all been reported to cause tubular disorders [3].

Under physiological conditions, albumin filtered by the glomerulus is reabsorbed in the tubules and urine albumin is detected at levels of 20 mg/g creatinine or less. In early DKD, however, tubular damage as well as glomerular damage cause increased urine albumin excretion, and this increase is used in clinical settings as the gold standard biomarker. Many observational studies have reported an association between albumin excreted in the urine and decreased glomerular filtration rate (GFR) [4, 5]. In the first half of the 1980s, 60–80% of diabetes patients with trace amounts of albumin in their urine had marked proteinuria after 6–14 years. However, recent research has found that 21–64% of these patients had gone into remission [6]. Thus, urine albumin cannot be used as a prognostic predictor for many DKD patients. These findings reflect the aggressive use of renin-angiotensin system inhibitors.

Nevertheless, there are reports that approximately 30% of type 2 diabetes patients with renal dysfunction do not have albuminuria [7] and that progressive glomerulosclerosis is detected on kidney biopsy in type 2 diabetes patients who do not have albuminuria [8]. Therefore, albuminuria and decreased kidney function are not necessarily correlated in at least some cases. Thus, there is a need for the development of a marker better than albuminuria for prognostic prediction and therapeutic response.

4.2.1.2 Tubular Damage Biomarkers

Urinary Neutrophil Gelatinase-Associated Lipocalin

Neutrophil gelatinase-associated lipocalin (NGAL) is a small molecule (25-kDa) that is released from tubular cells into the urine. This protein has been used in research as a biomarker for acute kidney injury [9–11]. In DKD, it is excreted in increasing amounts in urine before the advent of albuminuria. A concurrent increase in NGAL excretion and kidney injury molecule (KIM)-1 is reportedly associated with progressive pathology [12].

Urinary α-1-Microglobulin

α-1-Microglobulin (MG) is filtered by the glomerular bodies and reabsorbed by the proximal tubules, where it is metabolized. Thus, the amount excreted in urine increases with glomerular cell damage. Several studies on diabetes patients with normal levels of albumin in the urine have reported the use of α1-MG as a biomarker of early nephropathy [13, 14]. This biomarker is distinctive in being a relatively inexpensive option.

Urinary Kidney Injury Molecule-1

KIM-1 is a membrane protein located in proximal tubule cells. It is excreted in higher amounts in tubule cell injury and has been studied as a biomarker of acute kidney injury [15, 16]. Increased KIM-1 excretion in urine and decreased GFR are reportedly related, and KIM-1 is even excreted in higher amounts in the presence of glomerular hyperfiltration, which reflects the early pathophysiology of DKD [17, 18].

Urinary L-Type Fatty Acid Binding Protein

L-type fatty acid binding protein (L-FABP) is a carrier protein present in the proximal tubular cytoplasm. It is used as a biomarker of tubule injury and simultaneous acute kidney injury [19]. It can also be used as a predictive factor for progression to end-stage kidney failure and cardiovascular disease in chronic kidney disease patients. In Japan, L-FABP measurements are covered by insurance, making it a commonly used clinical test. As with the aforementioned biomarkers, L-FABP is excreted in higher amounts in diabetic urine despite normal albumin levels and is reportedly associated with DKD progression [20, 21].

Urinary Angiotensinogen

Urinary angiotensinogen reflects activation of the renin-angiotensin system localized in the kidneys. It is reportedly found in increased amounts in the urine of diabetes patients with normal urine albumin levels [22].

Urinary Cystatin C

Cystatin C (CysC) is a low-molecular-weight protein that is produced by all nucleated cells throughout the body. After filtration by the glomerular bodies, it is reabsorbed in the tubules. Urinary CysC is a biomarker of early nephropathy and is reportedly associated with simultaneous decline in renal function [23, 24]. Serum CysC is not affected by muscle mass, age, or sex and is used in clinical settings as a marker of early kidney dysfunction.

Urinary *N*-Acetyl-Glucosaminidase

N-Acetyl-glucosaminidase (NAG), an enzyme present in the proximal tubules, is a biomarker used to identify tubular disorders [25]. It is frequently used in clinical settings to differentiate nephropathy patients. Type 1 diabetes patients, who were the subjects of the Diabetes Control and Complications Trial, showed elevated urinary NAG at baseline. This elevated urinary NAG was found to be an independent risk factor for albuminuria during the 9-year observation period [26].

4.2.1.3 Glomerular Injury Biomarkers

Urinary Type IV Collagen

Type IV collagen is a constituent of the glomerular basement membrane and mesangial matrix. Increased excretion of type IV collagen in the urine is seen in early DKD and reflects structural changes in the glomerular bodies that are consistent with tissue changes [27]. Collagen excretion in the urine has a relatively high degree of specificity for DKD and thus is used to differentiate DKD from other forms of nephropathy.

Urinary Ceruloplasmin

Ceruloplasmin is a serum protein used in the transport of copper. As ceruloplasmin has a negative charge, it is not normally filtered by the glomerular bodies; as a result, it is utilized as a biomarker of glomerular disorders. It is reportedly found in increased levels in urine prior to the appearance of albuminuria [28].

Others

Other urinary substances that may have use as biomarkers of early DKD include transferrin, IgG, laminin, glycosaminoglycan, and lipocalin-type prostaglandin-D synthase.

4.2.2 Urinary and Serum Inflammatory Biomarkers

4.2.2.1 Inflammatory Cytokines

A variety of factors have been shown to contribute to the progression of DKD [29]. As chronic inflammation is one of these factors, all inflammatory cytokines can be used as biomarkers of DKD. Studies have reported that serum interleukin (IL)-6 levels become elevated in conjunction with increased excretion of albumin in the urine [30]. Baseline levels of IL-6, IL-8, monocyte chemoattractant protein (MCP)-1, and interferon-inducible protein (IP-10) in type 1 diabetes patients are reportedly higher in the urine of patients with early kidney damage [31].

Serum IL-18 levels are elevated from the early stage of DKD and studies have reported an association with cardiovascular death [32, 33].

Serum and urinary tumor necrosis factor-α (TNF-α) is reportedly elevated from the early stage of DKD [34], but serum TNF-α receptors may be more reflective of the pathophysiology of nephropathy [35].

4.2.2.2 Growth Factors

Transforming growth factor (TGF)-β regulates cell proliferation and differentiation and is one of the cytokines that is important for the maintenance of physiological homeostasis. Urinary TGF-β levels are elevated in DKD patients [36]. Recent study of type 2 diabetes patients has reported that the use of angiotensin-converting enzyme inhibitors or vitamin D causes urinary TGF-β levels to fall [37].

Connective tissue growth factor (CTGF) plays an important role in the body, similar to that of TGF. Urinary CTGF is closely associated with the excretion of albumin in the urine [38]. In type I diabetes patients, urinary CTGF is reportedly associated with both albuminuria and GFR [39]. Serum CTGF levels in type I diabetes patients are reportedly associated with end-stage kidney failure or mortality [40].

4.2.2.3 Adhesion Molecules

Elevated levels of serum intercellular adhesion molecule (ICAM)-1 are reportedly associated with albuminuria or the onset of trace amounts of albumin in the urine [41]. Serum vascular cell adhesion protein (VCAM)-1 and selectin have reportedly been associated with the pathophysiology of DKD [42], but as the data are conflicting, the use of these substances for assessment has not been established.

4.2.2.4 Other Factors

Fetuin-A is a vascular calcification inhibitor that is secreted by the liver. As kidney dysfunction progresses, serum levels decrease. In their study using a lectin microarray on urine samples from type 2 diabetes patients, Inoue et al. reported that fetuin-A could be used as a marker for microalbuminuria and decreased GFR [43].

CD40 ligands are expressed in B cells, antigen-presenting cells, and vascular endothelial cells. The soluble CD40 ligand is released during the activation of platelets, which allows its use as a marker for acute coronary syndrome. Serum soluble CD40 ligand is reportedly elevated before the onset of nephropathy [44].

Human $\alpha 1$ acid glycoprotein (orosomucoid), an acute reactant, is secreted in large amounts in the urine in nephrotic syndrome. This indicates the transition in diabetes patients from normal albumin levels in the urine to elevated urinary albumin levels [45].

4.2.3 Serum and Urinary Oxidative Stress Biomarkers

In both type 1 and type 2 diabetes patients, serum reactive oxygen species (e.g., oxidized low-density lipoprotein) levels are elevated, and antioxidant (e.g., superoxide dismutase, antioxidative vitamins, and bilirubin) levels are decreased [46, 47]. Urinary 8-oxo-7 and 8-dihydro-2′-deoxyguanosine (8-OHdG) are often used as oxidative stress markers. Patients with high amounts of urinary 8-OHdG reportedly have progressive DKD [48], but other reports have shown no association between the two; therefore, this substance has not been established for use in assessment. Pentosidine, a serum marker of oxidative stress, is reportedly an independent marker of microvascular lesions in type 2 diabetes patients [49]. By elevating oxidative stress levels and accelerating the renin-angiotensin system, uric acid promotes the progression of diabetic complications [50]. Therefore, this marker that can be utilized to evaluate pathophysiology and the therapeutic target.

4.2.4 *Development of Novel Biomarkers*

4.2.4.1 Integrated Omics Analysis in the Development of Comprehensive Biomarkers

Analytical Methods Using Metabolomics

The estimated number of metabolites in the human body ranges between 3000 and 8000. This number is vastly smaller than the approximate numbers of other omics in the body (genomics, 22,000; transcriptomics, 100,000; proteomics, 1 million).

However, there is no definitive method that can be used to analyze these metabolites simultaneously, as they all have differing chemical and physical properties. For example, it is almost impossible to simultaneously measure both hydrophilic metabolites, such as organic acids and nucleic acid bases, and hydrophobic metabolites such as fatty acids and phospholipids in a single analysis. In addition, as the number of possible metabolites ranges on the order of 10^7–10^9, collective analysis is even more unlikely. Therefore, metabolites are currently analyzed by first focusing only on those in the same metabolite group.

4.2.4.2 Application of Omics Analysis to the Development of Urinary Biomarkers of DKD (Table 4.2)

Proteomic Analysis

The Steno Diabetes Center reported on the results of urinary proteomic analysis using capillary electrophoresis coupled to mass spectrometry, which is highly

Table 4.2 Candidate biomarkers of diabetic nephropathy obtained from omics analysis

Omics analysis	Metabolome	miRNA		Integrated omics analysis
Biomarker candidate molecule	3-Indoxylsulfuric acid Glycerophospholipids Free fatty acids Tryptophan Uric acid Bile acids Organic anion transporters (OKT1, OKT3) Markers of mitochondrial metabolic dysfunction (PGC1α)	Increase	miRNA-377 miRNA-192 miRNA-216/217 miRNA-144 has-miR-453 has-miR-221 has-miR-524-5p has-miR-188-3p	MDM2 (MDM2 proto-oncogene, E3 ubiquitin protein ligase)
		Decrease	miRNA-21 miRNA-375 has-miR-214 has-miR-92b has-miR-765 has-miR-492 has-miR-373 has-miR-1913 has-miR-638	
References	[46, 47]	[48, 49]		[51–53]

reproducible. They could distinguish healthy individuals from diabetics by using 40 types of urinary peptide panels. Using an additional 65 types of peptides, they could also distinguish DKD as it progressed from the microalbuminuria phase to the overt proteinuria phase, which takes at least 3 years. Many of these were type 1 fragments [51]. In addition, the amounts of some of the 65 peptides that are excreted in the urine are known to decrease before the appearance of albuminuria, which makes them likely candidates for application in earlier diagnosis of DKD [52]. We believe that conducting comparisons of proteomic analysis profiles using the previously reported urinary biomarkers and panels shown in Fig. 4.1 is important.

Metabolomic Analysis

A number of molecules have been reported to be candidates for use in metabolomic analysis methods for DKD [53]. These are also important to the elucidation of the mechanism of DKD onset, but there are great hopes that they can additionally be used as biomarkers. Determining their clinical usefulness, however, remains a topic for future study.

Urinary metabolomic analysis using gas chromatography and mass spectrometry in combination has allowed researchers to identify profiles showing that decreases in the amounts of organic acids excreted in the urine, due to abnormalities in OKT1, OKT3, and other organic anion transporters, are more likely to occur in patients with DKD rather than in those without DKD [54]. We have also conducted metabolomic analyses using capillary electrophoresis-time-of-flight mass spectrometry on serum and urine samples collected from DKD patients at all stages of the disease.

We conducted statistical analysis of all peaks obtained. The results of principle component analysis, using all peaks found to have a significant difference from blood serum, indicated that although the separation of stage I and stage II was unclear, the results did allow us to determine that as the disease stages progressed, all sample plots showed a forward shift in the principle component. This suggests that the disease stage can be inferred from metabolomics data [55]. We obtained urinary metabolites with a positive or inverse correlation with albuminuria and

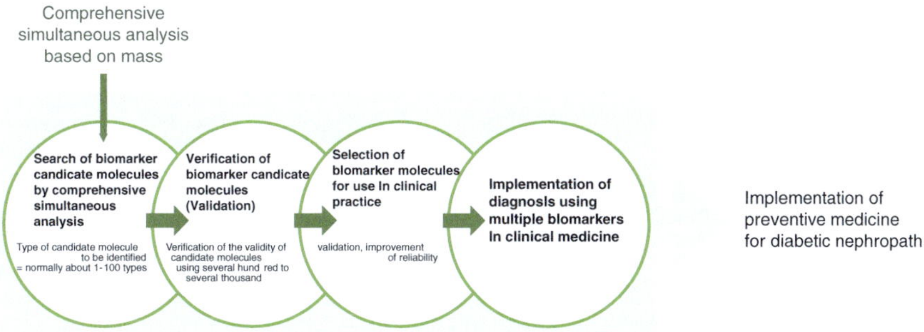

Fig. 4.1 Flowchart of development of diabetic nephropathy biomarkers

kidney function and are currently conducting assessments of unidentified and identified peaks, using these metabolites as biomarkers.

miRNA

Yang et al. confirmed that certain miRNAs (miRNA-377, miRNA-192, miRNA-216/217, miRNA-144) increase in the blood of DKD patients while others (miRNA-21, miRNA-375) decrease [56]. However, they found no correlation with kidney-specific urinary miRNAs. Argyropoulos et al. reported on urinary miRNA profiles that showed promise for use in the early diagnosis and prognostic prediction of nephropathy in type 1 diabetes patients [57]. These data may be useful in the further development of DKD urinary biomarker research.

4.2.4.3 Exploratory Biomarkers Identified by Research Performed by the Ministry of Health, Labour and Welfare (MHLW)/AMED Team (Representative: Takashi Wada)

The team led by Dr. Wada compiled the "Guide to Pathological Diagnosis of Diabetic Nephropathy" in 2015 and proposed the definition and scoring of pathological characteristics. This clarified the relationship between pathological findings characteristic of diabetic nephropathy and renal prognosis [58].

In meetings of the biomarker subcommittee, biomarkers in blood and urine, including known markers (L-FABP) approved domestically, have been proposed as exploratory markers (Fig. 4.2). The team has evaluated the utility of these biomarkers by analyzing their characteristics and forming panels. The team is working on

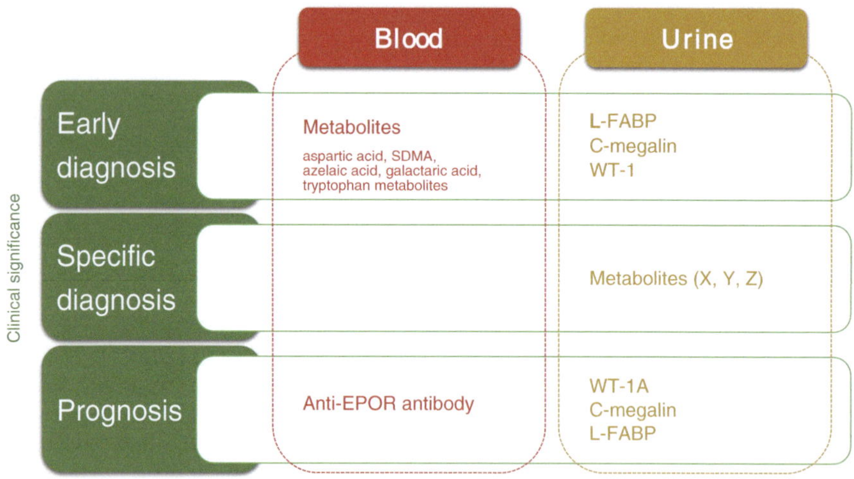

Fig. 4.2 Clinical significance of exploratory diabetic nephropathy biomarkers

the development of a diagnostic method that integrates pathological findings and biomarkers at each stage of diabetic nephropathy.

Metabolomic analysis has identified several metabolites in blood (e.g., aspartic acid, SMDA, azelaic acid, galactaric acid, tryptophan metabolites) and urine (e.g., L-FABP, C-megalin, and WT-1) as biomarkers for the early diagnosis of diabetic nephropathy.

Urinary metabolites (X, Y, and Z; patent pending) have been shown to diagnose for specific stages of diabetic nephropathy.

Several biomarkers were found to be prognostic of outcomes in patients with diabetic nephropathy. These include anti-erythropoietin receptor antibody and metabolites (e.g., tryptophan metabolites) in blood and L-FABP, A-megalin, WT-1, and metabolites in urine.

Analysis of the relationships between these biomarkers and characteristic pathological findings in patients with diabetic nephropathy utilized pathological specimens and urine samples collected by the Wada team. These analyses showed relationships between anti-erythropoietin receptor antibody and stromal cell invasion/interstitial fibrosis, between L-FABP and interstitial fibrosis and between tryptophan metabolites and stromal cell infiltration/full nodal sclerosis.

Testing of L-FABP is already covered by insurance. Assays for other biomarkers, including metabolites (e.g., aspartic acid, SMDA, azelaic acid, and galactaric acid), A-megalin and C-megalin, WT-1, and anti-erythropoietin receptor antibody, have been patented. WT-1 and anti-erythropoietin receptor antibodies are being prepared for clinical application, including their performance as in vitro diagnostic agents.

References

1. Macisaac RJ, Ekinci EI, Jerums G. Markers of and risk factors for the development and progression of diabetic kidney disease. Am J Kidney Dis. 2014;63(2 Suppl 2):S39–62.
2. Hohenstein B, Hausknecht B, Boehmer K, Riess R, Brekken RA, Hugo CP. Local VEGF activity but not VEGF expression is tightly regulated during diabetic nephropathy in man. Kidney Int. 2006;69(9):1654–61.
3. Vallon V, Komers R. Pathophysiology of the diabetic kidney. Compr Physiol. 2011;1(3):1175–232.
4. Newman DJ, Mattock MB, Dawnay AB, Kerry S, McGuire A, Yaqoob M, Hitman GA, Hawke C. Systematic review on urine albumin testing for early detection of diabetic complications. Health Technol Assess. 2005;9(30):iii–vi, xiii–163.
5. de Jong PE, Gansevoort RT. Albuminuria in non-primary renal disease: risk marker rather than risk factor. Nephrol Dial Transplant. 2010;25(3):656–8.
6. Macisaac RJ, Jerums G. Diabetic kidney disease with and without albuminuria. Curr Opin Nephrol Hypertens. 2011;20(3):246–57.
7. Kim SS, Song SH, Kim IJ, Kim WJ, Jeon YK, Kim BH, Kwak IS, Lee EK, Kim YK. Nonalbuminuric proteinuria as a biomarker for tubular damage in early development of nephropathy with type 2 diabetic patients. Diabetes Metab Res Rev. 2014;30(8):736–41.
8. Budhiraja P, Thajudeen B, Popovtzer M. Absence of albuminuria in type 2 diabetics with classical diabetic nephropathy: clinical pathological study. JBiSE. 2013;6:20–5.

9. Mishra J, Dent C, Tarabishi R, Mitsnefes MM, Ma Q, Kelly C, Ruff SM, Zahedi K, Shao M, Bean J, Mori K, Barasch J, Devarajan P. Neutrophil gelatinase-associated lipocalin (NGAL) as a biomarker for acute renal injury after cardiac surgery. Lancet. 2005;365(9466):1231–8.
10. Wheeler DS, Devarajan P, Ma Q, Harmon K, Monaco M, Cvijanovich N, Wong HR. Serum neutrophil gelatinase-associated lipocalin (NGAL) as a marker of acute kidney injury in critically ill children with septic shock. Crit Care Med. 2008;36(4):1297–303.
11. Constantin JM, Futier E, Perbet S, Roszyk L, Lautrette A, Gillart T, Guerin R, Jabaudon M, Souweine B, Bazin JE, Sapin V. Plasma neutrophil gelatinase-associated lipocalin is an early marker of acute kidney injury in adult critically ill patients: a prospective study. J Crit Care. 2010;25(1):176.e1–6.
12. de Carvalho JA, Tatsch E, Hausen BS, Bollick YS, Moretto MB, Duarte T, Duarte MM, Londero SW, Premaor MO, Comim FV, Delanghe JR, Moresco RN. Urinary kidney injury molecule-1 and neutrophil gelatinase-associated lipocalin as indicators of tubular damage in normoalbuminuric patients with type 2 diabetes. Clin Biochem. 2016;49(3):232–6.
13. Hong CY, Hughes K, Chia KS, Ng V, Ling SL. Urinary alpha1-microglobulin as a marker of nephropathy in type 2 diabetic Asian subjects in Singapore. Diabetes Care. 2003;26(2):338–42.
14. Petrica L, Petrica M, Vlad A, Jianu DC, Gluhovschi G, Ianculescu C, Firescu C, Dumitrascu V, Giju S, Gluhovschi C, Bob F, Gadalean F, Ursoniu S, Velciov S, Bozdog G, Milas O. Proximal tubule dysfunction is dissociated from endothelial dysfunction in normoalbuminuric patients with type 2 diabetes mellitus: a cross-sectional study. Nephron Clin Pract. 2011;118(2):c155–64.
15. Han WK, Bailly V, Abichandani R, Thadhani R, Bonventre JV. Kidney Injury Molecule-1 (KIM-1): a novel biomarker for human renal proximal tubule injury. Kidney Int. 2002;62(1):237–44.
16. Shao X, Tian L, Xu W, Zhang Z, Wang C, Qi C, Ni Z, Mou S. Diagnostic value of urinary kidney injury molecule 1 for acute kidney injury: a meta-analysis. PLoS One. 2014;9(1):e84131. https://doi.org/10.1371/journal.pone.0084131.
17. Bonventre JV. Kidney injury molecule-1 (KIM-1): a urinary biomarker and much more. Nephrol Dial Transplant. 2009;24(11):3265–8.
18. Fu WJ, Xiong SL, Fang YG, Wen S, Chen ML, Deng RT, Zheng L, Wang SB, Pen LF, Wang Q. Urinary tubular biomarkers in short-term type 2 diabetes mellitus patients: a cross-sectional study. Endocrine. 2012;41(1):82–8.
19. Kamijo-Ikemori A, Sugaya T, Obama A, Hiroi J, Miura H, Watanabe M, Kumai T, Ohtani-Kaneko R, Hirata K, Kimura K. Liver-type fatty acid-binding protein attenuates renal injury induced by unilateral ureteral obstruction. Am J Pathol. 2006;169(4):1107–17.
20. Kamijo-Ikemori A, Sugaya T, Yasuda T, Kawata T, Ota A, Tatsunami S, Kaise R, Ishimitsu T, Tanaka Y, Kimura K. Clinical significance of urinary liver-type fatty acid-binding protein in diabetic nephropathy of type 2 diabetic patients. Diabetes Care. 2011;34(3):691–6.
21. Nielsen SE, Sugaya T, Hovind P, Baba T, Parving HH, Rossing P. Urinary liver-type fatty acid-binding protein predicts progression to nephropathy in type 1 diabetic patients. Diabetes Care. 2010;33(6):1320–4.
22. Saito T, Urushihara M, Kotani Y, Kagami S, Kobori H. Increased urinary angiotensinogen is precedent to increased urinary albumin in patients with type 1 diabetes. Am J Med Sci. 2009;338(6):478–80.
23. Garg V, Kumar M, Mahapatra HS, Chitkara A, Gadpayle AK, Sekhar V. Novel urinary biomarkers in pre-diabetic nephropathy. Clin Exp Nephrol. 2015;19(5):895–900.
24. Kim SS, Song SH, Kim IJ, Jeon YK, Kim BH, Kwak IS, Lee EK, Kim YK. Urinary cystatin C and tubular proteinuria predict progression of diabetic nephropathy. Diabetes Care. 2013;36(3):656–61.
25. Parikh CR, Lu JC, Coca SG, Devarajan P. Tubular proteinuria in acute kidney injury: a critical evaluation of current status and future promise. Ann Clin Biochem. 2010;47(Pt 4):301–12.

26. Kern EF, Erhard P, Sun W, Genuth S, Weiss MF. Early urinary markers of diabetic kidney disease: a nested case-control study from the Diabetes Control and Complications Trial (DCCT). Am J Kidney Dis. 2010;55(5):824–34.
27. Okonogi H, Nishimura M, Utsunomiya Y, Hamaguchi K, Tsuchida H, Miura Y, Suzuki S, Kawamura T, Hosoya T, Yamada K. Urinary type IV collagen excretion reflects renal morphological alterations and type IV collagen expression in patients with type 2 diabetes mellitus. Clin Nephrol. 2001;55(5):357–64.
28. Narita T, Sasaki H, Hosoba M, Miura T, Yoshioka N, Morii T, Shimotomai T, Koshimura J, Fujita H, Kakei M, Ito S. Parallel increase in urinary excretion rates of immunoglobulin G, ceruloplasmin, transferrin, and orosomucoid in normoalbuminuric type 2 diabetic patients. Diabetes Care. 2004;27(5):1176–81.
29. Navarro-González JF, Mora-Fernández C, Muros de Fuentes M, García-Pérez J. Inflammatory molecules and pathways in the pathogenesis of diabetic nephropathy. Nat Rev Nephrol. 2011;7(6):327–40.
30. Saraheimo M, Teppo AM, Forsblom C, Fagerudd J, Groop PH. Diabetic nephropathy is associated with low-grade inflammation in Type 1 diabetic patients. Diabetologia. 2003;46(10):1402–7.
31. Wolkow PP, Niewczas MA, Perkins B, Ficociello LH, Lipinski B, Warram JH, Krolewski AS. Association of urinary inflammatory markers and renal decline in microalbuminuric type 1 diabetics. J Am Soc Nephrol. 2008;19(4):789–97.
32. Moriwaki Y, Yamamoto T, Shibutani Y, Aoki E, Tsutsumi Z, Takahashi S, Okamura H, Koga M, Fukuchi M, Hada T. Elevated levels of interleukin-18 and tumor necrosis factor-alpha in serum of patients with type 2 diabetes mellitus: relationship with diabetic nephropathy. Metabolism. 2003;52(5):605–8.
33. Szeto CC, Chow KM, Poon PY, Kwan BC, Li PK. Association of interleukin-18 promoter polymorphism and atherosclerotic diseases in Chinese patients with diabetic nephropathy. Nephrology (Carlton). 2009;14(6):606–12.
34. Navarro JF, Mora C, Maca M, Garca J. Inflammatory parameters are independently associated with urinary albumin in type 2 diabetes mellitus. Am J Kidney Dis. 2003;42(1):53–61.
35. Lopes-Virella MF, Baker NL, Hunt KJ, Cleary PA, Klein R, Virella G, DCCT/EDIC Research Group. Baseline markers of inflammation are associated with progression to macroalbuminuria in type 1 diabetic subjects. Diabetes Care. 2013;36(8):2317–23.
36. Riojas MA, Villanueva-Vedia RE, Zamilpa R, Chen X, Du LC, Phelix CF, LeBaron RG. Prevalence of diabetes mellitus and correlation of urinary transforming growth factor-beta1 with blood hemoglobin A1C in the Atascosa Diabetes Study. Ethn Dis. 2008;18(2 Suppl 2):S2–54–59.
37. Kim MJ, Frankel AH, Donaldson M, Darch SJ, Pusey CD, Hill PD, Mayr M, Tam FW. Oral cholecalciferol decreases albuminuria and urinary TGF-β1 in patients with type 2 diabetic nephropathy on established renin-angiotensin-aldosterone system inhibition. Kidney Int. 2011;80(8):851–60.
38. Gilbert RE, Akdeniz A, Weitz S, Usinger WR, Molineaux C, Jones SE, Langham RG, Jerums G. Urinary connective tissue growth factor excretion in patients with type 1 diabetes and nephropathy. Diabetes Care. 2003;26(9):2632–6.
39. Nguyen TQ, Tarnow L, Andersen S, Hovind P, Parving HH, Goldschmeding R, van Nieuwenhoven FA. Urinary connective tissue growth factor excretion correlates with clinical markers of renal disease in a large population of type 1 diabetic patients with diabetic nephropathy. Diabetes Care. 2006;29(1):83–8.
40. Nguyen TQ, Tarnow L, Jorsal A, Oliver N, Roestenberg P, Ito Y, Parving HH, Rossing P, van Nieuwenhoven FA, Goldschmeding R. Plasma connective tissue growth factor is an independent predictor of end-stage renal disease and mortality in type 1 diabetic nephropathy. Diabetes Care. 2008;31(6):1177–82.

41. Clausen P, Jacobsen P, Rossing K, Jensen JS, Parving HH, Feldt-Rasmussen B. Plasma concentrations of VCAM-1 and ICAM-1 are elevated in patients with Type 1 diabetes mellitus with microalbuminuria and overt nephropathy. Diabet Med. 2000;17(9):644–9.
42. Rubio-Guerra AF, Vargas-Robles H, Lozano Nuevo JJ, Escalante-Acosta BA. Correlation between circulating adhesion molecule levels and albuminuria in type-2 diabetic hypertensive patients. Kidney Blood Press Res. 2009;32(2):106–9.
43. Inoue K, Wada J, Eguchi J, Nakatsuka A, Teshigawara S, Murakami K, Ogawa D, Terami T, Katayama A, Tone A, Iseda I, Hida K, Yamada M, Ogawa T, Makino H. Urinary fetuin-A is a novel marker for diabetic nephropathy in type 2 diabetes identified by lectin microarray. PLoS One. 2013;8(10):e77118. https://doi.org/10.1371/journal.pone.0077118.
44. Chiarelli F, Giannini C, Verrotti A, Mezzetti A, Mohn A. Increased concentrations of soluble CD40 ligand may help to identify type 1 diabetic adolescents and young adults at risk for developing persistent microalbuminuria. Diabetes Metab Res Rev. 2008;24(7):570–6.
45. Jiang H, Guan G, Zhang R, Liu G, Liu H, Hou X, Cheng J. Increased urinary excretion of orosomucoid is a risk predictor of diabetic nephropathy. Nephrology (Carlton). 2009;14(3):332–7.
46. Chang CM, Hsieh CJ, Huang JC, Huang IC. Acute and chronic fluctuations in blood glucose levels can increase oxidative stress in type 2 diabetes mellitus. Acta Diabetol. 2012;49(Suppl 1):S171–7.
47. Whaley-Connell A, Sowers JR. Oxidative stress in the cardiorenal metabolic syndrome. Curr Hypertens Rep. 2012;14(4):360–5.
48. Hinokio Y, Suzuki S, Hirai M, Suzuki C, Suzuki M, Toyota T. Urinary excretion of 8-oxo-7, 8-dihydro-2′-deoxyguanosine as a predictor of the development of diabetic nephropathy. Diabetologia. 2002;45(6):877–82.
49. Kerkeni M, Saïdi A, Bouzidi H, Letaief A, Ben Yahia S, Hammami M. Pentosidine as a biomarker for microvascular complications in type 2 diabetic patients. Diab Vasc Dis Res. 2013;10(3):239–45.
50. Lytvyn Y, Perkins BA, Cherney DZ. Uric acid as a biomarker and a therapeutic target in diabetes. Can J Diabetes. 2015;39(3):239–46.
51. Rossing K, Mischak H, Dakna M, Zürbig P, Novak J, Julian BA, Good DM, Coon JJ, Tarnow L, Rossing P, Predictions Network. Urinary proteomics in diabetes and CKD. J Am Soc Nephrol. 2008;19:1283–90.
52. Zürbig P, Jerums G, Hovind P, Macisaac RJ, Mischak H, Nielsen SE, Panagiotopoulos S, Persson F, Rossing P. Urinary proteomics for early diagnosis in diabetic nephropathy. Diabetes. 2012;61:3304–13.
53. Weiss R, Kim K. Metabolomics in the study of kidney diseases. Nat Rev Nephrol. 2012;8:22–33.
54. Sharma K, Karl B, Mathew AV, Gangoiti JA, Wassel CL, Saito R, Pu M, Sharma S, You YH, Wang L, Diamond-Stanic M, Lindenmeyer MT, Forsblom C, Wu W, Ix JH, Ideker T, Kopp JB, Nigam SK, Cohen CD, Groop PH, Barshop BA, Natarajan L, Nyhan WL, Naviaux RK. Metabolomics reveals signature of mitochondrial dysfunction in diabetic kidney disease. J Am Soc Nephrol. 2013;24(11):1901–12.
55. Hirayama A, Nakashima E, Sugimoto M, Akiyama S, Sato W, Maruyama S, Matsuo S, Tomita M, Yuzawa Y, Soga T. Metabolic profiling reveals new serum biomarkers for differentiating diabetic nephropathy. Anal Bioanal Chem. 2012;404:3101–9.
56. Yang Y, Xiao L, Li J, Kanwar YS, Liu F, Sun L. Urine miRNAs:potential biomarkers for monitoring progression of early stages of diabetic nephropathy. Med Hypotheses. 2013;81:274–8.
57. Argyropoulos C, Wang K, McClarty S, Huang D, Bernardo J, Ellis D, Orchard T, Galas D, Johnson J. Urinary microRNA profiling in the nephropathy of type 1 diabetes. PLoS One. 2013;8:e54662.
58. Furuichi K, Yuzawa Y, Shimizu M, Hara A, Toyama T, Kitamura H, Suzuki Y, Sato H, Uesugi N, Ubara Y, Hisano S, Ueda Y, Nishi S, Yokoyama H, Nishino T, Kohagura K, Ogawa D, Mise K, Shibagaki Y, Kimura K, Haneda M, Makino H, Matsuo S, Wada T. Nationwide multicentre kidney biopsy study of Japanese patients with type 2 diabetes. Nephrol Dial Transplant. 2017;33(1):138–48. https://doi.org/10.1093/ndt/gfw417.

Chapter 5
Blood Pressure Management in Diabetic Kidney Disease

Naoki Kashihara

5.1 Introduction

Kidney disease is associated with a high risk of stroke and cardiovascular disease (CVD) prior to progression into end-stage kidney disease (ESKD) over many years. A disease concept known as chronic kidney disease (CKD) has been proposed considering the importance of early detection of kidney disease, which allows its early prevention and treatment.

In 2017 and 2018, major hypertension guidelines were revised worldwide. The latest guidelines in Japan are the Antihypertensive Therapy Guidelines 2019 (JSH 2019) issued by the Japanese Society of Hypertension [1] and the Evidence-Based CKD Treatment Guidelines 2018 (CKD Treatment GL 2018) of the Japanese Society of Nephrology [2]. Both were released around the same time. At a consensus conference held by the guideline committees of both societies, no conflicts arose regarding their frameworks. Consequently, they were able to maintain a high degree of consistency between the two sets of guidelines (Table 5.1).

From the early stage of the disease, patients with diabetic kidney disease (DKD) are at a high risk of CVD, which is a leading cause of ESKD in many countries.

Generally, the presence of microalbuminuria is an indicator to diagnose early-stage DKD. However, the risk of CVD is increased within the lower limit of the definition of microalbuminuria. The general rules for its prevention and treatment are (1) strict blood glucose level control, (2) strict blood pressure (BP) control, (3) optimization of abnormal metabolism such as lipid metabolism, and (4) optimization of body weight. If the appropriate treatment is provided, the onset and

N. Kashihara (✉)
Department of Nephrology and Hypertension, Kawasaki Medical School, Kurashiki, Okayama Prefecture, Japan
e-mail: kashinao@med.kawasaki-m.ac.jp

T. Wada et al. (eds.), *Diabetic Kidney Disease*,
https://doi.org/10.1007/978-981-15-9301-7_5

Table 5.1 JSH 2019 and CKD diagnostic and treatment guidelines

JSH 2019		Evidence-based CKD diagnosis and treatment guidelines 2018	
Diabetes (+)	BP under 130/80 mmHg	Diabetes complicating CKD All A classifications	BP under 130/80 mmHg is recommended
Diabetes (−) No proteinuria	BP under 140/90 mmHg	Diabetes non-complicating CKD All A classifications	Maintenance of BP under 140/90 mmHg is recommended
Proteinuria	BP under 130/80 mmHg	In classifications A2 and A3	Target BP under 130/80 mmHg is recommended

Proteinuria in JSH 2014: Proteinuria/urine creatinine ratio of at least 0.15 g/gCr

CKD diagnostic and treatment guidelines 2013, classification A2: Proteinuria/urine creatinine ratio of at least 0.15–0.49 g/gCr

Classification A3: Proteinuria/urine creatinine ratio of at least 0.5 g/gCr

BP blood pressure, *CKD* chronic kidney disease, *JSH 2019* Antihypertensive Therapy Guidelines 2019 issued by the Japanese Society of Hypertension

progression of DKD can be suppressed if optimal treatment is performed sufficiently. Remission and regression can be expected. Early diagnosis is crucial; therefore, measurement of microalbuminuria is essential.

5.2 Basic Strategy for CKD Treatment

The goal of CKD treatment, including that of DKD, is the prevention of stroke and CVD and the suppression of ESKD.

The three principles of antihypertensive therapy in CKD/DKD are (1) strict BP control over a 24-h period, (2) proper selection of antihypertensive drugs, and (3) reduction of albuminuria and proteinuria as much as possible.

It is important to understand the pathophysiology of DKD to implement appropriate antihypertensive therapy.

5.3 Basic Pathophysiology of DKD

5.3.1 Alterations in Microhemodynamics in the Kidney

Microhemodynamic changes and metabolic disorders in the kidney are involved in the development of DKD. The kidney is equipped with mechanisms that regulate the BP and microhemodynamics in the kidney to maintain homeostasis. In diabetes, this autoregulatory mechanism is impaired. Elevated intra-glomerular pressure (glomerular hypertension) is the characteristic change occurring in this condition. Since renal function (glomerular filtration ratio; GFR) is primarily determined by glomerular BP, it leads to an increase in GFR (hyperfiltration) [3]. Hyperfiltration is postulated to be the major mechanism for the development and progression of DKD (Fig. 5.1) [4]. Hyperfiltration can be treated in the early stage of DKD; however, it becomes more difficult to treat as the disease progresses.

Diabetes disrupts this homeostatic mechanism through multiple mechanisms: (1) tubuloglomerular feedback (TGF) mechanism, in which sodium resorption is increased via sodium-glucose co-transporter (SGLT), which is associated with increased resorption of glucose in the proximal tubules, followed by weakened afferent arteriole vascular resistance; (2) deterioration of the myogenic reaction caused by abnormalities in the functioning of the membrane-potential-dependent Ca channel; and (3) activation of the renin-angiotensin system [5]. Although diabetes is associated with a low renin state, the tissue renin-angiotensin system in the renal tissue is paradoxically promoted [6]. This activation of the RA system leads to a convergence of insulin resistance and activation of the sympathetic nervous system (Fig. 5.2).

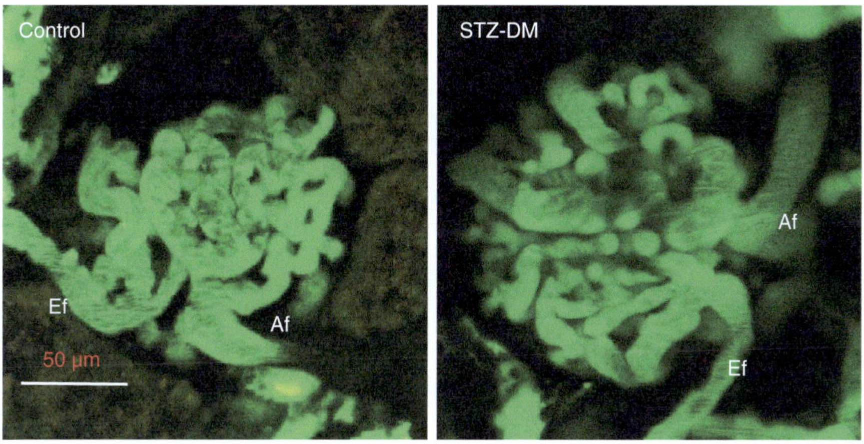

Fig. 5.1 Structural changes in the glomeruli in diabetes. Streptozotocin-induced diabetes rat model after 4 weeks, 50× magnification. In the early stages of diabetes, the afferent arterioles dilate, the efferent arterioles contract, and the glomeruli enlarge. When FITC-labeled dextran is administered to diabetic rats, the blood flow becomes visible, and the use of a two-photon laser microscope has allowed observation of the glomeruli in living kidneys in real time [4]. *Af* afferent arterioles, *Ef* efferent arterioles, *STZ-DM* streptozotocin-induced diabetes mellitus. Using this method, we investigated the structural changes in diabetic glomeruli. The image shown here is of a STZ-DM onset glomerulus at 5 weeks and the control glomerulus. Compared to the glomerulus of the control rat, The STZ-DM rat glomerulus shows increased overall size. In addition, compared to the efferent artery of the STZ-DM rat, the afferent artery is relatively dilated

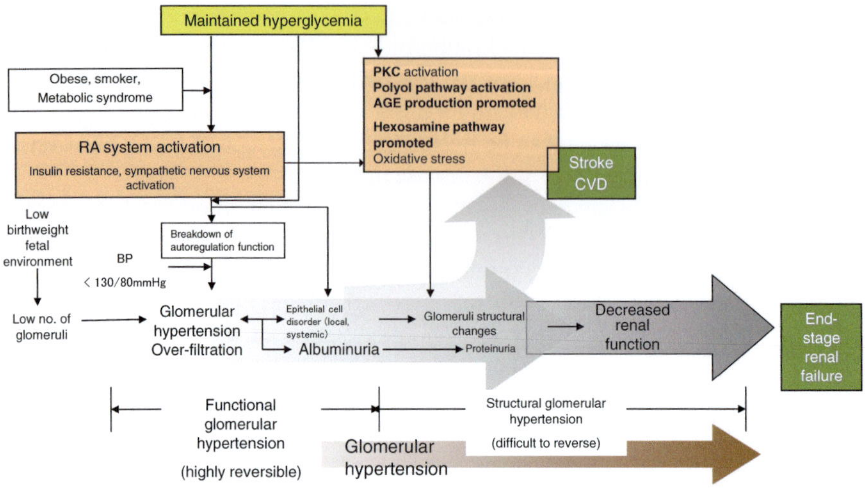

Fig. 5.2 The mechanism of diabetic kidney disease onset and progression. The pathophysiology of the onset and progression of diabetic kidney disease involves two basic mechanisms: (1) abnormal intra-renal hemodynamics (intra-glomerular hypertension) and (2) metabolic abnormalities caused by hyperglycemia. Once the autoregulation function of the afferent arterioles breaks down, intra-glomerular pressure becomes dependent upon systemic BP; consequently, it becomes necessary to reduce BP to under 130/80 mmHg. When glomerular hypertension and endothelial (functional) disorder occur concurrently, albuminuria develops. This then progresses into proteinuria, which in turn leads to renal failure. Initially, the "functional" glomerular hypertension is highly reversible, but as structural changes in the glomeruli progress, there is a shift to "structural" glomerular hypertension, which is more difficult to treat

5.3.2 Vascular Endothelial Dysfunction

In diabetes, vascular endothelial dysfunction develops during the early stages of the disease. Nitric oxide synthase (NOS), which is an NO-producing enzyme, exhibits both oxidation and reduction ability. When coenzyme BH4 is insufficient, the electrons produced by NADPH oxidation are provided to the oxygen molecules, following which NOS starts to produce O^{2-} (uncoupling). Satoh et al. observed that in the glomeruli of diabetic mice, O^{2-} is produced not only by NAD(P)H oxidase but also by NOS [7, 8]. They determined that this was caused by eNOS uncoupling caused by a decrease in coenzyme BH4. Additionally, the administration of BH4 has been shown to ameliorate urinary excretion of albumin [9].

5.4 BP Management in DKD

In the presence or absence of kidney complications, the BP for diabetes patients is recommended to be maintained under 130/80 mmHg. Most clinical studies that investigated the effectiveness of antihypertension therapies for patients with diabetes have not shown actual achievement of the target BP under 130/80 mmHg;

therefore, there is little basis for the effectiveness of strictly lowering the BP to this extent.

The ACCORD-BP trial [10] demonstrated no effectiveness in the prevention of CVD in the group with strictly lowered BP (mean BP achieved was 119.3/64.4 mmHg) compared to that in the group with conventionally lowered BP (133.5/70.5 mmHg); however, there was an increase in serious adverse events. There was, however, a significantly lower incidence of stroke—which is common in Japan—in the group with strictly lowered BP. Additionally, this group exhibited significantly lower proteinuria levels. The impetus for the present study was the results from a meta-study of 13 trials indicating that patients with diabetes were successful in lowering BP to below 135/80 mmHg, which was consistent with this result [11]. Additionally, analysis of decreased proteinuria determined that strictly lowering BP was effective in this regard. Based on these results, the guidelines recently released in Europe and the United States were revised so that they now recommend the BP target to be under 140/80–85 mmHg.

Nevertheless, unlike Europe and the United States, it has been shown by the Hisayamamachi Study [12] and the Suita Study [13] that, in Japan, stroke onset is far more prevalent than ischemic heart disease or myocardial infarction. In consideration of these differences, the target BP in patients with diabetes in Japan is determined by JSH 2019 to be under 130/80 mmHg.

The JSH 2019 and the CKD treatment GL 2018 recommend the following BP targets:

1. In cases of diabetes:

    (a) Under 130/80 mmHg, regardless of whether albuminuria is present or not

2. In cases of CKD without diabetes:

    (a) Proteinuria (−): Under 140/90 mmHg
    (b) Proteinuria (+): Under 130/80 mmHg

In cases of CKD without diabetes, when the proteinuria status is (−) according to the dipstick test, there is little evidence indicating the effectiveness of strict BP control under 130/80 mmHg for the prevention of CVD and ESKD [14].

5.5 First-Line Treatment for DKD

In cases of diabetic hypertension, the recommended first-line antihypertensive drug treatment was previously RA inhibitors, regardless of whether DKD is present or not. RA inhibitors are also recommended for patients with hypertension due to their possible inhibitory effect on the development of type 2 diabetes in these patients. These recommendations were primarily based on a sub-analysis of clinical trials and preclinical studies [15].

However, recent analyses showed no difference in efficacy among the three classes of antihypertensive drugs, RA inhibitors, Ca channel blockers, and diuretics, in populations with diabetes. Thus, the latest guidelines recommend these three classes equally for the first-line treatment of hypertensive patients with diabetes.

In cases complicated with DKD, RA inhibitors are recommended as the first-line drug, at least at the microalbuminuria stage (recommendation grade of A).

5.5.1 *Effectiveness of RA Inhibitors in Inhibiting Progression of DKD*

Multiple clinical studies have shown that RA inhibitors are effective in the inhibition of DKD progression in both type 1 and type 2 diabetes.

The following results are obtained from a typical large-scale clinical study targeting early nephropathy due to type 2 diabetes (second stage).

In the IRMA-2 study, the angiotensin II receptor blocker (ARB) irbesartan significantly suppressed urinary albumin excretion (UAE) [16]. Forty-nine patients in the placebo group progressed from microalbuminuria to overt nephropathy with proteinuria, while in the irbesartan 150 mg group and 300 mg group, this ratio was suppressed to 9.7% and 5.2%, respectively. Progression was suppressed in a dose-dependent manner. Additionally, the INNOVATION study focused on early-stage nephropathy; it included Japanese subjects with normal BP. In contrast to the placebo group, in which 44.2% patients transitioned to overt proteinuria, in the telmisartan 40 mg and 80 mg groups, this percentage was suppressed to 21.0% (NNT 3.66) and 11.9% (NNT 3.01), respectively [17].

Even in the overt proteinuria stage (third stage), the renal protective action of RA inhibitors has been verified. The RENAAL study targets advanced diabetic nephropathy with serum creatinine 1.9 mg/dL. Compared to the placebo, the losartan group exhibited a 16% reduction in the composite endpoint, which consisted of doubling of serum creatinine, end-stage renal failure, and death. Sub-analyses have also shown a positive correlation between the rate of urinary protein decrease and renal prognosis [18]. In the IDNT study, irbesartan suppressed the progression of renal damage. The ORIENT study using olmesartan showed that the rate of GFR decline was delayed; simultaneously, it demonstrated the inhibitory effect of olmesartan on cardiovascular events [19].

Furthermore, there are racial differences in the effects of RA inhibitors; these effects become apparent in Asians, especially the Japanese [20].

5.5.2 *Preventive Effect of RA Inhibitors Against DKD*

It has been suggested that RA inhibitors may suppress not only the progression of nephropathy but also the onset. The BENEDICT study, which targeted patients with type 2 diabetes along with hypertension, demonstrated that the angiotensin-converting enzyme (ACE) inhibitor trandolapril was able to inhibit the onset of microalbuminuria [16].

In contrast, in studies on normotensive type 1 diabetes, losartan administration accelerated the onset of microalbuminuria [21]. The average HbA1c in this study was high at 8.6%, indicating poor glycemic control. However, the BP was normal at 120/70 mmHg. ARB could not suppress the onset of nephropathy in normotensive type 1 diabetes, where blood sugar control is poor. Contrarily, in the BENEDICT study, which targeted patients with type 2 diabetes and hypertension (average BP of 150/87 mmHg), the average HbA1c was 5.8%, indicating good blood glucose control.

There are two explanations for the contrast between these results. RA system inhibitors dilate the afferent arterioles and increase renal blood flow; however, this effect is often overlooked because their effect on efferent arterioles is emphasized. As a result, the GFR increases in healthy individuals [22]. Type 1 diabetes does not involve insulin resistance. The afferent arterioles dilate in a blood-glucose-dependent manner in the early stage of diabetes. Therefore, RA inhibitors may increase albuminuria in type 1 diabetes. In addition to the difference between type 1 and type 2 diabetes, differences in the control status for blood glucose and BP in these studies may contribute to the difference in these results.

5.6 Antihypertensive Drug Combination Therapy

RA inhibitors are utilized as the first-line drug for hypertension; however, when they do not sufficiently lower of BP, combination therapy with second-line drugs such as long-acting Ca antagonist, thiazide diuretics (including thiazide-like drugs such as CKD G1–G3), and loop diuretics (CKD G4–G5) is considered. Combination therapy with RA inhibitors and small doses of diuretics may achieve a major decrease in proteinuria; however, decreased GFR is also common. If the decrease in GFR is less than 30% of the previous value, the long-term prognosis of renal function is good. In fact, in clinical trials of RA inhibitors for DKD, most patients were administered RA inhibitors in combination with small doses of diuretics [23].

5.6.1 The Advantages of Combination Therapy with an RA Inhibitor and Diuretic

Patients with DKD often present salt-sensitive hypertension. Salt sensitivity is a cause of nocturnal hypertension (such as in a non-dipper). Nocturnal BP is usually 10–20% lower than daytime, waking BP (dipper). The risk of stroke, CVD, and cognitive impairment is higher in the riser type, which is associated with an increase in nocturnal BP, and the non-dipper type. Additionally, non-dipper type nocturnal hypertension is a risk factor for developing albuminuria. Diuretics are excellent in correcting nocturnal BP abnormalities.

Since diuretics reduce the renal blood flow, they activate the RA system. This promotes the vascular resistance of the efferent arterioles, which in turn function as a "safety valve" that maintains intra-glomerular pressure and preserves the GFR. In cases in which diuretics and RA inhibitors are used in combination, the RA system does not function as a safety valve when the amount of body fluid decreases. This subsequently makes it difficult to maintain the GFR. Although the combination of RA inhibitors and diuretics increases the effectiveness of proteinuria suppression, the GFR is considerably decreased for this reason. In elderly individuals and others, the risk of hyponatremia is increased.

Additionally, limiting salt intake enhances the organ-protective effects of RA inhibitors. Among the participants in the RENAAL and IDNT trials, results have been reported from the analyses of patients who were able to undergo 24-h urine collection. When the salt intake values were divided into three quartiles, the ARB-treated group exhibited the lowest incidence of renal and cardiovascular events in the group with the lowest salt intake.

The GUARD study compared the effects of the combination of the ACE inhibitor benazepril + amlodipine with the combination of benazepril + hydrochlorothiazide in patients with type 2 diabetes exhibiting hypertension and albuminuria. The patients were randomly assigned to two groups in a double-blind fashion. The primary endpoint was albuminuria after 52 weeks. The observation period was 1 year.

The observed antihypertensive effect was the same in both groups. Although in both groups, the urinary albumin excretion compared with the baseline value significantly decreased, it was −72.1% in the hydrochlorothiazide combination group and 40.5% in the amlodipine combination group. The former group exhibited a greater reduction in albuminuria ($P < 0.0001$) [24].

Changes in the eGFR, which were analyzed as a secondary outcome, were −2.03 ± 14.2 mL/min/1.73 m^2 in the amlodipine combination group and −13.64 ± 16.1 mL/min/1.73 m^2 in the hydrochlorothiazide combination group ($P < 0.0001$); the eGFR was significantly maintained in the amlodipine combination group.

Conflicting results were obtained between the two groups, with respect to the proteinuria reduction effect and the GFR retention ability. It remains unclear whether the combinations of RA inhibitors with diuretics and RA inhibitors with Ca antagonists can improve the prognosis of renal function.

5.6.2 *The Advantages of Combination Therapy with Ca Antagonist*

The L-type Ca channel is widely distributed in the intra-renal vascular system up to the efferent arterioles. Generally, dihydropyridine Ca antagonists (calcium channel blocker; CCB), all of which act on the L-type Ca channel, are used. CCBs increase the renal blood flow and increase the effective glomerular filtration area. Since they increase the blood flow in the peritubular capillaries, they act to suppress Na resorption (diuretic effect) and relieve interstitial ischemia. These effects are beneficial as they protect the kidneys.

However, some clinical studies have reported that they are weaker at reducing proteinuria than RA inhibitors or that they increase proteinuria. In contrast, CCB administration in non-CKD hypertension patients does not cause proteinuria. Additionally, in the elderly, it has been shown to gradually improve the GFR [25]. The clinical studies that found that CCB administration is not beneficial in terms of renal protection have one point in common; in all of them, the subjects were CKD patients who presented a minimum level of proteinuria. Specifically, in cases with glomerular hypertension (proteinuria), the results suggest that CCB administration may further increase proteinuria.

Therefore, when CCBs are used in CKD patients who present proteinuria at a certain level or higher, then the following conditions should be met: (1) a long-acting CCB should be selected (low activation of the sympathetic nervous system), (2) sufficient lowering of the BP should be achieved (arterial pressure is more easily transmitted to intra-glomerular pressure), and (3) a subclass (T-type, N-type, types that do not markedly activate the sympathetic nervous system) that can be expected to dilate the efferent arterioles should be selected.

In case of patients such as the elderly (low renal blood flow) and patients with arteriosclerotic nephrosis, CCBs are the first-line drug as their advantages are mostly manifested in such cases. CCBs are an extremely safe option for the kidneys because, when they are used on the types of cases indicated above, they are not associated with unexpected acute renal dysfunction.

5.6.3 Combination Therapy with RA Inhibitors

It has been established that RA inhibitors possess an excellent ability to reduce proteinuria. Indeed, that effectiveness has been shown to be considerably more dependent upon the dose of the RA inhibitor than the degree to which the BP is lowered; thus, sufficient doses (high doses) are recommended when the goal is to reduce proteinuria.

The combined use of RA inhibitors with different mechanisms of action (double blockade) can be expected to produce, in theory, a comprehensive RA inhibitory effect and, therefore, a more additive and synergistic organ-protective effect.

To conclusively verify the efficacy of the combination therapy, large-scale, international, multicenter, joint, double-blind studies have been conducted. However, contrary to the expectations, these extensive studies did not show that combined therapy was effective. Besides, they showed an increased risk of adverse events [26, 27].

5.7 Conclusion

Hypertension in DKD patients is an important factor that determines prognosis. Appropriate BP management—specifically, the setting of appropriate BP targets and the selection of appropriate antihypertensive drugs—is important. It has been shown that if strict BP management and sufficient blood glucose management can be utilized at least until the microalbuminuria stage, remission induction can be expectantly achieved without nephropathy onset or progression. However, nephropathy experienced as a complication in patients with diabetes has various clinical presentations, all of which fall under the rubric of DKD. In addition to following the guidelines, individualized medical care should be implemented.

References

1. Umemura S, Arima H, Arima S, et al. The Japanese Society of Hypertension Guidelines for the Management of Hypertension (JSH 2019). Hypertens Res. 2019;42:1235–481.
2. Okada H, Research Team for a Grant-in-Aid for Research on Advanced Chronic Kidney Disease, Practical Research Project for Renal Diseases from Japan Agency for Medical Research, et al. Essentials from clinical practice guidelines for CKD stage G3b-5 2017. Clin Exp Nephrol. 2018;22:245–8.
3. Kashihara N, Haruna Y, Kondeti VK, et al. Oxidative stress in diabetic nephropathy. Curr Med Chem. 2010;17:4256–69.
4. Satoh M, Kobayashi S, Kuwabara A, et al. In vivo visualization of glomerular microcirculation and hyperfiltration in streptozotocin-induced diabetic rats. Microcirculation. 2010;17:103–12.
5. Parving HH, Kastrup H, Smidt UM, et al. Impaired autoregulation of glomerular filtration rate in type 1 (insulin-dependent) diabetic patients with nephropathy. Diabetologia. 1984;27:547–52.
6. Ichihara A, Kaneshiro Y, Takemitsu T, et al. The (pro)renin receptor and the kidney. Semin Nephrol. 2007;27:524–8.
7. Satoh M, Fujimoto S, Haruna Y, et al. NAD(P)H oxidase and uncoupled nitric oxide synthase are major sources of glomerular superoxide in rats with experimental diabetic nephropathy. Am J Physiol Renal Physiol. 2005;288:F1144–52.
8. Satoh M, Fujimoto S, Arakawa S, et al. Angiotensin II type 1 receptor blocker ameliorates uncoupled endothelial nitric oxide synthase in rats with experimental diabetic nephropathy. Nephrol Dial Transplant. 2008;23:3806–13.
9. Kidokoro K, Satoh M, Channon KM, et al. Maintenance of endothelial guanosine triphosphate cyclohydrolase I ameliorates diabetic nephropathy. J Am Soc Nephrol. 2013;24:1139–50.
10. Group Accord Study, Group Accord Eye Study Group, Chew EY, et al. Effects of medical therapies on retinopathy progression in type 2 diabetes. N Engl J Med. 2010;363:233–44.
11. Bangalore S, Kumar S, Lobach I, et al. Blood pressure targets in subjects with type 2 diabetes mellitus/impaired fasting glucose: observations from traditional and bayesian random-effects meta-analyses of randomized trials. Circulation. 2011;123:2799–810.
12. Arima H, Anderson C, Omae T, et al. Effects of blood pressure lowering on major vascular events among patients with isolated diastolic hypertension: the perindopril protection against recurrent stroke study (PROGRESS) trial. Stroke. 2011;42:2339–41.
13. Kokubo Y, Kamide K, Okamura T, et al. Impact of high-normal blood pressure on the risk of cardiovascular disease in a Japanese urban cohort: the Suita study. Hypertension. 2008;52:652–9.

14. Rahman M, Ford CE, Cutler JA, et al. Long-term renal and cardiovascular outcomes in Antihypertensive and Lipid-Lowering Treatment to Prevent Heart Attack Trial (ALLHAT) participants by baseline estimated GFR. Clin J Am Soc Nephrol. 2012;7:989–1002.
15. Jandeleit-Dahm KA, Tikellis C, Reid CM, et al. Why blockade of the renin-angiotensin system reduces the incidence of new-onset diabetes. J Hypertens. 2005;23:463–73.
16. Andersen S, Brochner-Mortensen J, Parving HH, et al. Kidney function during and after withdrawal of long-term irbesartan treatment in patients with type 2 diabetes and microalbuminuria. Diabetes Care. 2003;26:3296–302.
17. Makino H, Haneda M, Babazono T, et al. Prevention of transition from incipient to overt nephropathy with telmisartan in patients with type 2 diabetes. Diabetes Care. 2007;30:1577–8.
18. Brenner BM, Cooper ME, de Zeeuw D, et al. Effects of losartan on renal and cardiovascular outcomes in patients with type 2 diabetes and nephropathy. N Engl J Med. 2001;345:861–9.
19. Imai E, Chan JC, Ito S, et al. Effects of olmesartan on renal and cardiovascular outcomes in type 2 diabetes with overt nephropathy: a multicentre, randomised, placebo-controlled study. Diabetologia. 2011;54:2978–86.
20. Kurokawa K, Chan JC, Cooper ME, et al. Renin angiotensin aldosterone system blockade and renal disease in patients with type 2 diabetes: a subanalysis of Japanese patients from the RENAAL study. Clin Exp Nephrol. 2006;10:193–200.
21. Ruggenenti P, Fassi A, Ilieva AP, et al. Preventing microalbuminuria in type 2 diabetes. N Engl J Med. 2004;351:1941–51.
22. Hollenberg NK, Fisher ND. Renal circulation and blockade of the renin-angiotensin system. Is angiotensin-converting enzyme inhibition the last word? Hypertension. 1995;26:602–9.
23. Esnault VL, Ekhlas A, Delcroix C, et al. Diuretic and enhanced sodium restriction results in improved antiproteinuric response to RAS blocking agents. J Am Soc Nephrol. 2005;16:474–81.
24. Bakris GL, Toto RD, McCullough PA, et al. Effects of different ACE inhibitor combinations on albuminuria: results of the GUARD study. Kidney Int. 2008;73:1303–9.
25. Suzuki H, Saruta T. Effects of calcium antagonist, benidipine, on the progression of chronic renal failure in the elderly: a 1-year follow-up. Clin Exp Hypertens. 2001;23:189–201.
26. Investigators Ontarget, Yusuf S, Teo KK, et al. Telmisartan, ramipril, or both in patients at high risk for vascular events. N Engl J Med. 2008;358:1547–59.
27. Parving HH, Brenner BM, McMurray JJ, et al. Cardiorenal end points in a trial of aliskiren for type 2 diabetes. N Engl J Med. 2012;367:2204–13.

Chapter 6
Glycemic Control and Future Perspectives for Treatment

Satoshi Miyamoto and Kenichi Shikata

6.1 Glycemic Control

6.1.1 Introduction

Diabetic kidney disease (DKD) is a well-known chronic pathological condition that develops and progresses as a result of long-term changes in glucose metabolism. DKD is one of the three major complications of diabetes, together with retinopathy and neuropathy.

Several factors are involved in the development of DKD, including increased polyol pathway flux, activation of protein kinase C, oxidative stress, accumulation of advanced glycation end products, glomerular hyperfiltration, overexpression of transforming growth factor-β (TGF-β), followed by increase of extracellular matrices. These mechanisms can act independently or in combination, leading to functional and histological abnormalities of the kidney in DKD patients. Chronic inflammation induced by the above mechanisms also plays a crucial role in the progression of DKD [1]. Since hyperglycemia is the most important contributing factor for DKD, glycemic control is important for suppression of the progression of nephropathy, improvement of patient prognosis, and reduction of medical costs.

In DKD patients, the mortality associated with cardiovascular diseases increases with an increase in albuminuria and deterioration of renal function (cardiorenal connection) [2]. American Diabetes Association's *Standards of Medical Care in Diabetes* (2020) [3] recommends that urinary albumin to creatinine ratio and eGFR should be measured at least once per year for patients with at least 5 years of type 1 diabetes and all patients with type 2 diabetes. The prognosis of DKD patients developing ESRD and requiring dialysis is poor. Therefore, in clinical practice, regular

S. Miyamoto · K. Shikata (✉)
Center for Innovative Clinical Medicine, Okayama University Hospital, Okayama, Japan
e-mail: shikata@md.okayama-u.ac.jp

T. Wada et al. (eds.), *Diabetic Kidney Disease*,
https://doi.org/10.1007/978-981-15-9301-7_6

screening of renal function is important because early diagnosis and appropriate early treatment of DKD are essential for preventing the progression of nephropathy in diabetes.

This chapter reviews evidences suggesting the effects of glycemic control on the prevention of the development and progression of DKD.

6.1.2 Glycemic Control and Prevention of Development and Progression of DKD

The following six randomized controlled trials (RCTs) examining the effects of strict glycemic control on the clinical outcomes, including subanalyses and follow-up analyses after trial completion, were reviewed: the Diabetes Control and Complications Trial (DCCT) [4–6] for type 1 diabetes patients, UK Prospective Diabetes Study (UKPDS) for type 2 diabetes patients, Kumamoto study [7], Action to Control Cardiovascular Risk in Diabetes (ACCORD) trial [8, 9], Action in Diabetes and Vascular Disease: Preterax and Diamicron Modified Release Controlled Evaluation (ADVANCE) trial [10–12], and Veterans Affairs Diabetes Trial (VADT) [13, 14].

DCCT [4] was an RCT involving 1441 patients with type 1 diabetes and a mean observation period of 6.5 years. The patients were randomly assigned to either an intensive insulin therapy group (target HbA1c < 6.05%, receiving insulin injections at least three times a day or use of an insulin pump) or a conventional therapy group. The results showed that intensive therapy reduced the risk of microalbuminuria (defined as urinary albumin excretion ≥ 40 mg/24 h) by 39% and that of albuminuria (defined as urinary albumin excretion ≥ 300 mg/24 h) by 54%. The Epidemiology of Diabetes Interventions and Complications (EDIC) study was conducted as a follow-up of DCCT. In EDIC, both groups received intensive insulin therapy. The results showed that despite the HbA1c levels were similar between the two groups, the rates of progression of albuminuria [15] and decrease in glomerular filtration rate (GFR) [5] were significantly lower in the group which had previously received the intensive insulin therapy with strict glycemic control, suggesting the importance of early strict glycemic control.

Besides DCCT and EDIC, the Kumamoto study [7], ADVANCE trial [10], ACCORD trial [8], and VADT [13] reported that strict glycemic control significantly prevented the development of microalbuminuria. The DCCT [4], Kumamoto study [7], ADVANCE trial [10], and ACCORD trial [8] reported that strict glycemic control significantly prevented the progression to macroalbuminuria. Furthermore, the ADVANCE trial [10] reported that strict glycemic control significantly reduced albuminuria and increased the rate of regression to normoalbuminuria (urinary albumin-creatinine ratio < 30 μg/mg). A meta-analysis of RCTs involving type 2 diabetes patients aged 19 years or older also revealed that compared to standard therapy, intensive therapy (median HbA1c during the study period was 6.4–7.4%) decreased the risks of both microalbuminuria and macroalbuminuria [16]. Thus, the results of multiple RTCs and meta-analysis suggest that strict glycemic control is effective for preventing the development and progression of DKD.

However, the results of RCTs suggesting the effects of strict glycemic control on prevention of the progression to ESRD remain controversial. The ADVANCE trial investigated type 2 diabetes patients with cardiovascular risk factors and reported that compared to standard therapy, intensive therapy (target HbA1c $\leq$ 6.5%) significantly reduced the risk of ESRD (requiring renal replacement therapy) by 65% [10]. On the other hand, DCCT/EDIC [5], ACCORD [8], and UKPDS33 [17] reported no significant difference in the risk of ESRD between the intensive therapy and standard therapy groups.

6.1.3 Relationship Between Strict Glycemic Control and Cardiovascular Events and Mortality

The ACCORD trial investigated type 2 diabetes patients with cardiovascular disease or cardiovascular risk factors and reported in 2008 that intensive therapy (target HbA1c < 6%) significantly increased mortality compared to the standard therapy (target HbA1c 7–7.9%) [18]. Subsequent analyses were conducted by dividing the subjects into those with and without CKD [CKD was defined as any of the following: (1) eGFR $\geq$ 90 mL/min/1.73 m^2 and urinary albumin/Cr ratio $\geq$ 30 μg/mg, (2) 60 $\leq$ eGFR $\leq$ 89 mL/min/1.73 m^2 and urinary albumin/Cr ratio $\geq$ 30 μg/mg, or (3) 30 $\leq$ eGFR $\leq$ 59 mL/min/1.73 m^2] [9]. The results of the analyses showed that intensive therapy significantly decreased the incidence of nonfatal myocardial infarction (hazard ratio [HR] = 0.74, 95% confidence interval [CI] = 0.59–0.93, p = 0.009) but significantly increased all-cause mortality (HR = 1.306; 95% CI = 1.065–1.600, p = 0.01) and cardiovascular death (HR = 1.412, 95% CI = 1.052–1.892, p = 0.02) in CKD patients; however, non-CKD patients showed no significant differences in all-cause mortality or cardiovascular death between the two groups.

On the other hand, results of the ADVANCE trial [11] (target HbA1c $\leq$ 6.5%) showed no significant difference in mortality between the two therapy groups, based on the analysis using the following two different cutoff points for CKD: (1) eGFR $\geq$ 60 and UACR $\geq$ 30 mg/g Cr and (2) eGFR < 60. The UKPDS post-trial monitoring study [19] (UKPDS80; median follow-up period, 16.8 years) and DCCT/EDIC [6] (mean follow-up period, 27 years) reported that the risk of all-cause mortality significantly decreased during the follow-up period in patients who had been treated with strict glycemic control; however, the subanalysis of CKD or DKD patients was not performed. On the other hand, the follow-up study of the VADT [14] (median follow-up period, 9.8 years) reported that strict glycemic control decreased the risk of major cardiovascular events, but there was no significant effect on all-cause mortality. Furthermore, a meta-analysis, involving the ACCORD trial, reported no significant difference in mortality between the standard and intensive therapy groups [20].

Thus, findings regarding the effect of strict glycemic control on all-cause mortality and cardiovascular events are inconsistent. Currently, the evidence is insufficient for the effect of glycemic control, especially in DKD patients.

6.1.4 Target Level of Glycemic Control and Points of Attention

Based on the findings of the Kumamoto study [21] and other RCTs [4, 12, 17], a target HbA1c level of <7% is recommended for prevention of the development and progression of microvascular complications including DKD. The *Standards of Medical Care in Diabetes (2020)* [22] recommends a target HbA1c level of <7% for diabetes patients and also proposes a target HbA1c level of <6.5% for preventing microvascular complications in patients whose blood glucose levels can be controlled without complications such as hypoglycemia. It is also suggested that the target HbA1c level can be set at <8% in patients with a history of severe hypoglycemia, limited life expectancy, and/or advanced micro- or macrovascular complications [23].

The DCCT [4], ADVANCE trial [12], VADT [13], and UKPDS33 [17] reported that strict glycemic control increased the incidence of severe hypoglycemia. Subanalysis of the ACCORD trial [9] results involving diabetes patients with CKD reported that the incidence of hypoglycemia requiring assistance was significantly higher in CKD patients than in non-CKD patients, and the annual incidence was 5.3% in CKD patients receiving intensive therapy, 2.0% in CKD patients receiving standard therapy, 3.5% in the non-CKD patients receiving intensive therapy, and 1.1% in the non-CKD patients receiving standard therapy. Therefore, careful blood glucose management considering the patient background and risks of hypoglycemia is needed, especially for patients with DKD with decreased eGFR because they are susceptible to hypoglycemia.

Furthermore, elderly patients tend to experience few symptoms at the time of hypoglycemia and, therefore, are susceptible to severe hypoglycemia due to strict glycemic control depending on the drugs used. In addition, patients with dementia and/or those with impaired activities of daily living may have problems such as difficulty in self-management. Thus, the target HbA1c level for each patient should be determined after a comprehensive assessment including risk of hypoglycemia, life expectancy, severity of vascular complications, and compliance [24].

DKD patients often have diabetic retinopathy. Assessment of retinopathy is mandatory when treatment for glycemic control is initiated. Treatment for retinopathy should be performed in parallel with that for glycemic control and in collaboration with ophthalmologists, if needed. Caution should be exercised while initiating treatment without confirming the presence of retinopathy, since there is a risk of exacerbating retinopathy if rapid glycemic control is performed [25]. DCCT [26] showed that progression of retinopathy was more common in the strict glycemic control group than in the standard therapy group at 6 and 12 months of the study; however, a reverse result was obtained thereafter. After 3.5 years, the development and progression of retinopathy was less common in the intensive insulin therapy group.

6.1.5 Glycemic Control in Patients with Renal Dysfunction

The importance of glycemic control in DKD patients with renal dysfunction has not been clearly established due to lack of sufficient evidence. Compared to patients with normal renal function, those with renal dysfunction have various problems including decreased gluconeogenesis in the kidney, decreased metabolism and excretion of insulin due to renal dysfunction, increased insulin resistance due to uremia, and other pharmacokinetic changes. In general, HbA1c is used as an index of glycemic control. However, besides HbA1c, glycoalbumin and blood glucose levels should also be used as glycemic control indices because patients with renal dysfunction may require treatment for renal anemia with erythropoietin, iron supplements, and/or infusion, all of which can reduce the red blood cell life span and increase immature erythrocytes, thereby reducing the HbA1c levels [27].

There is insufficient evidence related to the efficacy of glycemic control in preventing the progression of DKD. A study on diabetes patients with stage G3 and G4 CKD reported that mortality and the incidence of end-stage renal failure and cardiovascular events increased with an increase in HbA1c levels and that mortality increased even in patients with HbA1c levels <6.5% [28].

A study of glycemic control in patients on hemodialysis reported that those with HbA1c levels >8.5% had higher mortality [23].

6.1.6 Intensive Therapy

The effects of intensive therapy on prevention of cardiovascular complications were demonstrated by the Steno-2 study conducted at the Steno Diabetes Center in Denmark. The Steno-2 study was an RCT examining the effects of multifactorial intensive therapy consisting of strict glycemic control and lifestyle intervention by a multidisciplinary team comprising physicians, nurses, and dieticians in 160 patients with type 2 diabetes and microalbuminuria. The intensive therapy group received comprehensive treatment including lifestyle intervention, strict glycemic and blood pressure control, serum lipid control, administration of angiotensin-converting enzyme (ACE) inhibitor or angiotensin receptor blocker (ARB), administration of supplements such vitamins C and E, and administration of aspirin. The progression of diabetic vascular complications, including DKD, was compared between the intensive therapy and standard therapy groups.

After a mean of 3.8 years of intervention, compared to the standard therapy group, the rate of progression of nephropathy (urinary albumin > 300 mg/24 h) was reduced by 73%, and the rates of retinopathy and autonomic disorder were reduced by 55% and 68%, respectively, in the intensive therapy group [29]. After a mean of 7.8 years of intervention, the incidence of composite cardiovascular events was significantly reduced by 53% in the intensive therapy group compared to the standard group [30]. During the observation period after completion of the trial, the prior standard therapy group also received intensive therapy. At a mean follow-up of 13.3 years, risk factors such as HbA1c level, low-density lipoprotein cholesterol level, and systolic blood pressure were not significantly different between the two groups; however, all-cause mortality and risks of cardiovascular death and cardiovascular events were reduced by 46%, 57%, and 59%, respectively, in the intensive therapy group [31]. The incidence of end-stage renal disease was also significantly decreased in the intensive therapy group compared to the standard group [31].

After a mean follow-up of 21.2 years [32], all-cause mortality was reduced by approximately 45% in the intensive therapy group, and the difference in median survival time was 7.9 years. In addition, the time to onset of first cardiovascular event was 8.1 years longer in the intensive therapy group. In the intensive therapy group, the rates of progression of diabetic microvascular complications (except peripheral neuropathy) were reduced, and the rate of progression of nephropathy was reduced by 48%.

Thus, while treating DKD, multifactorial intensive intervention including glycemic control, blood pressure control using the renin–angiotensin system inhibitor, lipid management, and diet therapy is considered important for the prevention of cardiovascular events, reduction of all-cause mortality, and prevention of end-stage renal disease. In order to effectively perform such intensive therapies in clinical practice, a multidisciplinary team comprising physicians, nurses, pharmacists, and dieticians is extremely important.

6.1.7 Conclusion

In clinical practice, maintaining appropriate blood glucose levels in diabetes is important for the prevention of neuropathy, and regular monitoring of urinary albumin and eGFR levels is important for the early diagnosis and treatment of nephropathy. Intensive therapy is necessary for DKD patients to not only prevent the progression of nephropathy and end-stage renal disease but also to reduce cardiovascular events and all-cause mortality.

6.2 Future Perspectives for Treatment

6.2.1 Introduction

Treatment of diabetic kidney disease (DKD) mainly consists of glycemic control, blood pressure control including suppression of the renin–angiotensin system (RAS), lipid control, and dietary therapy. Until recently, the angiotensin-converting enzyme (ACE) inhibitor and angiotensin receptor blocker (ARB) are the only drugs that had been proven to be effective for treating DKD. Since DKD is the most common cause of end-stage renal disease (ESRD), development of new drugs for DKD is an urgent need.

Hyperglycemia is the most important contributing factor in the progression of DKD. Besides hyperglycemia, hypertension and dyslipidemia are also involved in the development and progression of DKD. Furthermore, multiple downstream mechanisms are considered to be involved in the development of DKD, and these mechanisms are of special interest in the development of new drugs.

This chapter reviews recent developments related to DKD therapeutics and focuses on new drugs which have been developed based on the factors involved in the pathogenesis of DKD.

6.2.2 Pathogenetic Factors for DKD

DKD is a renal disease induced by chronic hyperglycemia. Many factors are considered to be involved in the disease progression/pathogenesis from the onset of hyperglycemia to development of glomerular sclerosis and interstitial fibrosis. There are several mechanisms downstream of hyperglycemia. These include activation of RAS and changes in glomerular hemodynamics, increased levels of cytokines (such as TGF-β), oxidative stress, accumulation of advanced glycation end products (AGEs) due to increased Maillard reaction, increased activation of protein kinase C (PKC) via abnormal intracellular metabolism (such as polyol metabolism abnormalities), and cell cycle abnormalities. In addition, chronic low-grade inflammation (microinflammation) in the renal tissue plays an important role as an accelerating factor for DKD.

6.2.2.1 Glycation Reaction

In diabetic patients, the non-enzymatic glycation reaction (Maillard reaction) is activated and AGEs accumulate in the body. As a result, macrophage activation and increased production of extracellular matrix from mesangial cells are induced via receptors for advanced glycation end products (RAGE) on macrophages and mesangial cells. In addition, accumulation of extracellular matrix is accelerated because it becomes resistant to enzymatic degradation after modification by AGEs. Recently, a trial of pyridoxamine, an AGE inhibitor, for DKD treatment was conducted.

6.2.2.2 Activation of RAS and Changes in Glomerular Hemodynamics

In diabetic patients, the afferent and efferent glomerular arterioles are dilated. It is assumed that intraglomerular pressure increases because the dilatation of afferent glomerular arterioles is greater than that of efferent glomerular arterioles. The RAS in the kidney is activated in diabetic patients, and angiotensin II induces glomerular hypertension by contracting the efferent glomerular arterioles.

It is also known that angiotensin II promotes proliferation of mesangial cells and proximal tubular cells and stimulates the production of TGF-β. It also stimulates macrophage accumulation and promotes inflammation via the production of chemokines such as monocyte chemoattractant protein-1 (MCP-1). Thus, activation of RAS in the kidney induces glomerular sclerosis and interstitial fibrosis via various mechanisms.

At present, the endothelin A receptor antagonist [33, 34] and mineralocorticoid receptor antagonist (described later) are under development for the treatment of DKD.

6.2.2.3 Abnormal Intracellular Metabolism

When a large amount of glucose is transported into the cells in a hyperglycemic state, the amount of glucose processed via the glucose metabolism pathways (polyol pathway, diacylglycerol [DAG] signaling pathway, and hexosamine biosynthetic pathway), except for the glycolytic pathways, increases, leading to sorbitol and DAG accumulation in the cells. Increased renal DAG content activates PKC, further leading to the activation of MAP kinase followed by increase in TGF-β expression. In an experiment using an animal model, a PKC-β inhibitor was reported to be effective in preventing the progression of DKD [35].

6.2.2.4 Oxidative Stress

Hyperglycemia promotes oxidative stress through increased activation of nicotinamide adenine dinucleotide phosphate (NADPH) oxidase and decreased activation of superoxide dismutase (SOD) which scavenges reactive oxygen species. In addition, the formation of Amadori rearrangement products and AGEs due to glycation leads to the generation of many reactive oxygen species. Furthermore, macrophages infiltrating the renal tissue generate free radicals. A trial of bardoxolone methyl, an antioxidant, for DKD treatment is currently underway (described later).

6.2.2.5 Inflammation

The expression of intercellular adhesion molecule-1 (ICAM-1) and chemokines (such as monocyte chemoattractant protein-1, MCP-1) and macrophage infiltration increase in the renal tissue of diabetic patients in a similar manner as that in the arterial sclerotic lesions [1]. In addition, the concentrations of various pro-inflammatory cytokines increase in the blood and urine of type 2 diabetes patients. The blood and urine concentrations of interleukin-18 (IL-18, a pro-inflammatory cytokine) positively correlate with urine albumin excretion [36]. The blood concentration of IL-18 also positively correlates with intima–media thickness (IMT) and brachial-ankle pulse wave velocity (baPWV), which are indices of arteriosclerosis [36]. Thus, recent studies validated that microinflammation, mainly caused by infiltrated macrophages, plays an important role in the pathogenesis of DKD. Recently, it was suggested that microinflammation is induced by the activation of inflammasome. It is also known that inflammation of visceral fat plays a role in the pathogenesis of insulin resistance associated with obesity, the central component of metabolic syndrome [37, 38].

Studies investigating the efficacy of DKD treatment by targeting inflammation have been performed. We conducted a study for examining the effects of statins and pioglitazone using a diabetic rat model and reported that these drugs were effective in suppressing macrophage infiltration and urinary albumin excretion and preventing the progression of glomerular fibrosis without influencing glucose metabolism and hemodynamics [1]. As described later, the GLP-1 receptor agonist, an incretin-related drug, has renal protective as well as antihyperglycemic effect.

6.2.3 *Therapeutics for DKD*

6.2.3.1 GLP-1 Receptor Antagonist

The GLP-1 receptor antagonist exerts an antihyperglycemic effect by promoting insulin secretion from pancreatic beta cells and suppressing glucagon secretion from pancreatic alpha cells. Given that GLP-1 receptors are expressed in various organs other than the pancreas, there is a possibility that the GLP-1 receptor agonist binds to these receptors to mediate this effect. Although there is no firm consensus about the sites of expression of GLP-1 receptor, recent studies have demonstrated that GLP-1 has various effects, including the vasodilatory and anti-inflammatory effects, besides the antihyperglycemic effect. We demonstrated in vitro that exenatide exerts an anti-inflammatory effect by decreasing the expression of ICAM-1 in glomerular endothelial cells [39]. We also conducted a study using type 1 diabetes model rats and reported that administration of exenatide improved oxidative stress, inflammation, and glomerular hyperfiltration in the renal tissue and reduced albuminuria and histological damage [39]. In the Liraglutide Effect and Action In Diabetes: Evaluation of Cardiovascular Outcome Results (LEADER) trial [40], administration of liraglutide significantly suppressed the nephropathy-related outcomes (onset of macroalbuminuria, doubling of the serum creatinine level and eGFR $\leq$ 45 mL/min/1.73 m^2, need for continuous renal replacement therapy, or death from renal disease) and has received much attention. The Trial to Evaluate Cardiovascular and Other Long-term Outcomes with Semaglutide in Subjects with Type 2 Diabetes (SUSTAIN-6) [41] also reported that administration of semaglutide significantly suppressed the nephropathy-related outcomes (persistent macroalbuminuria, persistent doubling of the serum creatinine level and a creatinine clearance of $\leq$45 mL/min/1.73 m^2 of body surface area, or need for continuous renal replacement therapy).

6.2.3.2 SGLT2 Inhibitor

SGLT2 inhibitors show hypoglycemic effects by increasing glucose excretion from the kidney. The Empagliflozin Cardiovascular Outcome Event Trial in Type 2 Diabetes Mellitus Patients-Removing Excess Glucose (EMPA-REG OUTCOME) [42, 43] trial examined the effects of empagliflozin on cardiovascular outcomes in type 2 diabetes patients with a history of cardiovascular disease. The results showed that empagliflozin significantly reduced cardiovascular endpoints. Notably, the treatment also reduced renal events (secondary endpoints). Furthermore, the Canagliflozin Cardiovascular Assessment Study (CANVAS) program [44] recently reported that compared to placebo, canagliflozin treatment significantly reduced the composite cardiovascular outcome (cardiovascular death, nonfatal myocardial infarction, or nonfatal stroke; primary outcome) in type 2 diabetes patients with cardiovascular disease or cardiovascular risk factors. In addition, canagliflozin also prevented the progression of albuminuria (increase of $\geq$30% or progression of disease stage) and composite renal outcome (40% decrease in eGFR, renal replacement therapy or renal disease-related death). Dapagliflozin is also reported to reduce the kidney events in DECLARE-TIMI 58 randomized trial [45].

A global clinical trial of canagliflozin for DKD treatment (Canagliflozin and Renal Endpoints in Diabetes with Established Nephropathy Clinical Evaluation; CREDENCE) [46] has been conducted. In this trial, canagliflozin reduced the relative risk of the renal-specific composite of end-stage kidney disease, a doubling of the creatinine level, or death from renal causes was lower by 34% [47]. These results suggest that SGLT2 inhibitor is beneficial for DKD.

6.2.3.3 Bardoxolone Methyl

Nuclear factor erythroid 2-related factor 2 (Nrf2) is a transcription factor that controls the expression of genes that modulate oxidative stress. The transcription of Nrf2 is controlled by Keap1, a sensor molecule. The Nrf2–Keap1 pathway is involved in maintaining homeostasis by sensing oxidative stress in the body and inducing defense reactions. Nrf2 plays an extremely important role in reducing oxidative stress and chronic inflammation. Regulating the defense mechanism against oxidative stress via Nrf2 activation is important for renal protection [48].

Bardoxolone methyl is a compound developed as a small molecule Nrf2 activator. It binds to Keap1 and facilitates nuclear translocation of Nrf2 by releasing the inhibition of Keap1 on Nrf2 [49]. In addition, it suppresses the activation of NF-κB by binding to IκB kinase [50]. The renal protective effect of bardoxolone methyl was observed when the drug was under development as an anticancer drug. Since then, the drug has been studied as a potent therapeutic agent for treating renal dysfunction. In the Bardoxolone Methyl Treatment: Renal Function in CKD/Type 2 Diabetes (BEAM) trial (phase II trial), 227 patients with type 2 diabetes and eGFR level of 20–45 mL/min/1.73 m^2 were treated with bardoxolone methyl or placebo for 52 weeks. A significant increase in eGFR was observed, as compared with placebo, at 24 and 52 weeks after treatment [51]. In the subsequent Bardoxolone Methyl Evaluation in Patients with Chronic Kidney Disease and Type 2 Diabetes Mellitus: the Occurrence of Renal Events (BEACON) trial (phase III trial), 2185 type 2 diabetes patients with eGFR level of 15–30 mL/min/1.73 m^2 were treated with bardoxolone methyl (20 mg/day) or placebo, and ESRD and death from cardiovascular causes were employed as the primary endpoints. However, the trial was discontinued after 9 months because of safety concerns, driven primarily by an increase in cardiovascular events [52].

In Japan, a phase II trial of bardoxolone methyl for DKD patients (the Phase II Study of Bardoxolone Methyl in Patients with Chronic Kidney Disease and Type 2 Diabetes; TSUBAKI trial) reported that a significant increase in GFR measured by inulin clearance was observed in the treatment group (according to the report released by Kyowa Hakko Kirin Co., Ltd. in May 2016). The drug is expected to have a renal protective effect that is different from those of conventional drugs, since it does not improve albuminuria. The results of clinical studies are awaited.

6.2.3.4 Mineralocorticoid Receptor Antagonist

Aldosterone is secreted by the adrenal gland in response to stimulation by angiotensin II. Therefore, aldosterone secretion can be suppressed by ACE inhibitor or ARB. However, long-term use of ACE inhibitor or ARB leads to a failure to suppress aldosterone levels in some patients (aldosterone breakthrough). The aldosterone breakthrough can be corrected by administration of spironolactone, a mineralocorticoid receptor (MR) antagonist, by which albuminuria is reduced.

A clinical trial of finerenone, a nonsteroidal MR antagonist, for DKD was conducted [53]. This double-blind trial examined the combinational effect of finerenone in DKD patients receiving ACE inhibitor or ARB. The results showed that additional administration of finerenone significantly reduced albuminuria, and there was no significant change in eGFR, with lower incidence of hyperkalemia. The systolic blood pressure was reduced by only approximately 5 mmHg even at the maximum dose of finerenone, suggesting that the effect of finerenone on albuminuria reduction was not associated with any hypotensive effect. Recently, it has been reported that adding esaxerenone on RAS inhibitor reduces urinary albumin-to-creatinine ratio in Japanese patients with type 2 diabetes and microalbuminuria [54].

6.2.4 Conclusions

This chapter reviewed therapeutic strategies for DKD treatment based on its pathogenesis and current status of new drug development for DKD. The prognosis and quality of life of diabetes patients can be improved by prevention of renal failure and cardiovascular death. This is achieved by preventing the development and progression of DKD with reduction or remission of albuminuria. In order to accomplish this, early diagnosis and treatment of albuminuria is important. Further, development of new drugs for treating early nephropathy in patients with microalbuminuria is urgent.

References

1. Shikata K, et al. Microinflammation in the pathogenesis of diabetic nephropathy. J Diabetes Investig. 2013;4:142–9.
2. Adler AI, et al. Development and progression of nephropathy in type 2 diabetes: the United Kingdom Prospective Diabetes Study (UKPDS 64). Kidney Int. 2003;63:225–32.
3. American Diabetes Association. 11. Microvascular complications and foot care: standards of medical care in diabetes-2020. Diabetes Care. 2020;43:S135–51.
4. Nathan DM, et al. The effect of intensive treatment of diabetes on the development and progression of long-term complications in insulin-dependent diabetes mellitus. N Engl J Med. 1993;329:977–86.
5. DCCT/EDIC Research Group, et al. Intensive diabetes therapy and glomerular filtration rate in type 1 diabetes. N Engl J Med. 2011;365:2366–76.
6. Writing Group for the DCCT/EDIC Research Group, et al. Association between 7 years of intensive treatment of type 1 diabetes and long-term mortality. JAMA. 2015;313:45–53.
7. Shichiri M, et al. Long-term results of the Kumamoto Study on optimal diabetes control in type 2 diabetic patients. Diabetes Care. 2000;23(Suppl 2):B21–9.
8. Ismail-Beigi F, et al. Effect of intensive treatment of hyperglycaemia on microvascular outcomes in type 2 diabetes: an analysis of the ACCORD randomised trial. Lancet. 2010;376:419–30.
9. Papademetriou V, et al. Chronic kidney disease and intensive glycemic control increase cardiovascular risk in patients with type 2 diabetes. Kidney Int. 2015;87:649–59.
10. Perkovic V, et al. Intensive glucose control improves kidney outcomes in patients with type 2 diabetes. Kidney Int. 2013;83:517–23.
11. Wong MG, et al. Long-term benefits of intensive glucose control for preventing end-stage kidney disease: ADVANCE-ON. Diabetes Care. 2016;39:694–700.
12. ADVANCE Collaborative Group, et al. Intensive blood glucose control and vascular outcomes in patients with type 2 diabetes. N Engl J Med. 2008;358:2560–72.
13. Duckworth W, et al. Glucose control and vascular complications in veterans with type 2 diabetes. N Engl J Med. 2009;360:129–39.

14. Hayward RA, et al. Follow-up of glycemic control and cardiovascular outcomes in type 2 diabetes. N Engl J Med. 2015;372:2197–206.
15. The Diabetes Control and Complications Trial/Epidemiology of Diabetes Interventions and Complications Research Group, et al. Retinopathy and nephropathy in patients with type 1 diabetes four years after a trial of intensive therapy. N Engl J Med. 2000;342:381–9.
16. Coca SG, et al. Role of intensive glucose control in development of renal end points in type 2 diabetes mellitus: systematic review and meta-analysis intensive glucose control in type 2 diabetes. Arch Intern Med. 2012;172:761–9.
17. Intensive blood-glucose control with sulphonylureas or insulin compared with conventional treatment and risk of complications in patients with type 2 diabetes (UKPDS 33). UK Prospective Diabetes Study (UKPDS) Group. Lancet. 1998;352:837–53.
18. Action to Control Cardiovascular Risk in Diabetes Study Group, et al. Effects of intensive glucose lowering in type 2 diabetes. N Engl J Med. 2008;358:2545–59.
19. Holman RR, et al. 10-year follow-up of intensive glucose control in type 2 diabetes. N Engl J Med. 2008;359:1577–89.
20. Boussageon R, et al. Effect of intensive glucose lowering treatment on all cause mortality, cardiovascular death, and microvascular events in type 2 diabetes: meta-analysis of randomised controlled trials. BMJ. 2011;343:d4169.
21. Ohkubo Y, et al. Intensive insulin therapy prevents the progression of diabetic microvascular complications in Japanese patients with non-insulin-dependent diabetes mellitus: a randomized prospective 6-year study. Diabetes Res Clin Pract. 1995;28:103–17.
22. American Diabetes Association. 6. glycemic targets: standards of medical care in diabetes-2020. Diabetes Care. 2020;43:S66–76.
23. Hill CJ, et al. Glycated hemoglobin and risk of death in diabetic patients treated with hemodialysis: a meta-analysis. Am J Kidney Dis. 2014;63:84–94.
24. Inzucchi SE, et al. Management of hyperglycemia in type 2 diabetes, 2015: a patient-centered approach: update to a position statement of the American Diabetes Association and the European Association for the Study of Diabetes. Diabetes Care. 2015;38:140–9.
25. Early worsening of diabetic retinopathy in the Diabetes Control and Complications Trial. Arch Ophthalmol. 1998;116:874–86.
26. The effect of intensive diabetes treatment on the progression of diabetic retinopathy in insulin-dependent diabetes mellitus. The Diabetes Control and Complications Trial. Arch Ophthalmol. 1995;113:36–51.
27. Inaba M, et al. Glycated albumin is a better glycemic indicator than glycated hemoglobin values in hemodialysis patients with diabetes: effect of anemia and erythropoietin injection. J Am Soc Nephrol. 2007;18:896–903.
28. Shurraw S, et al. Association between glycemic control and adverse outcomes in people with diabetes mellitus and chronic kidney disease: a population-based cohort study. Arch Intern Med. 2011;171:1920–7.
29. Gæde P, et al. Intensified multifactorial intervention in patients with type 2 diabetes mellitus and microalbuminuria: the Steno type 2 randomised study. Lancet. 1999;353:617–22.
30. Gæde P, et al. Multifactorial intervention and cardiovascular disease in patients with type 2 diabetes. N Engl J Med. 2003;348:383–93.
31. Gæde P, et al. Effect of a multifactorial intervention on mortality in type 2 diabetes. N Engl J Med. 2008;358:580–91.
32. Gæde P, et al. Years of life gained by multifactorial intervention in patients with type 2 diabetes mellitus and microalbuminuria: 21 years follow-up on the Steno-2 randomised trial. Diabetologia. 2016;59:2298–307.
33. Schievink B, et al. Prediction of the effect of atrasentan on renal and heart failure outcomes based on short-term changes in multiple risk markers. Eur J Prev Cardiol. 2016;23:758–68.
34. Heerspink HJL, et al. Atrasentan and renal events in patients with type 2 diabetes and chronic kidney disease (SONAR): a double-blind, randomised, placebo-controlled trial. Lancet. 2019;393:1937–47.

35. Koya D, et al. Characterization of protein kinase C beta isoform activation on the gene expression of transforming growth factor-beta, extracellular matrix components, and prostanoids in the glomeruli of diabetic rats. J Clin Invest. 1997;100:115–26.
36. Nakamura A, et al. Serum interleukin-18 levels are associated with nephropathy and atherosclerosis in Japanese patients with type 2 diabetes. Diabetes Care. 2005;28:2890–5.
37. Kanda H, et al. MCP-1 contributes to macrophage infiltration into adipose tissue, insulin resistance, and hepatic steatosis in obesity. J Clin Invest. 2006;116:1494–505.
38. Kamei N, et al. Overexpression of monocyte chemoattractant protein-1 in adipose tissues causes macrophage recruitment and insulin resistance. J Biol Chem. 2006;281:26602–14.
39. Kodera R, et al. Glucagon-like peptide-1 receptor agonist ameliorates renal injury through its anti-inflammatory action without lowering blood glucose level in a rat model of type 1 diabetes. Diabetologia. 2011;54:965–78.
40. Marso SP, et al. Liraglutide and cardiovascular outcomes in type 2 diabetes. N Engl J Med. 2016;375:311–22.
41. Marso SP, et al. Semaglutide and cardiovascular outcomes in patients with type 2 diabetes. N Engl J Med. 2016;375:1834–44.
42. Zinman B, et al. Empagliflozin, cardiovascular outcomes, and mortality in type 2 diabetes. N Engl J Med. 2015;373:2117–28.
43. Wanner C, et al. Empagliflozin and progression of kidney disease in type 2 diabetes. N Engl J Med. 2016;375:323–34.
44. Neal B, et al. Canagliflozin and cardiovascular and renal events in type 2 diabetes. N Engl J Med. 2017;377:644–57.
45. Mosenzon O, et al. Effects of dapagliflozin on development and progression of kidney disease in patients with type 2 diabetes: an analysis from the DECLARE-TIMI 58 randomised trial. Lancet Diabetes Endocrinol. 2019;7:606–17.
46. Jardine MJ, et al. The canagliflozin and renal endpoints in diabetes with established nephropathy clinical evaluation (CREDENCE) study rationale, design, and baseline characteristics. Am J Nephrol. 2017;46:462–72.
47. Perkovic V, et al. Canagliflozin and renal outcomes in type 2 diabetes and nephropathy. N Engl J Med. 2019;380:2295–306.
48. Suzuki T, et al. Stress-sensing mechanisms and the physiological roles of the Keap1-Nrf2 system during cellular stress. J Biol Chem. 2017;292:16817–24.
49. Zoja C, et al. The Nrf2 pathway in the progression of renal disease. Nephrol Dial Transplant. 2014;29(Suppl 1):i19–24.
50. Ahmad R, et al. Triterpenoid CDDO-Me blocks the NF-kappaB pathway by direct inhibition of IKKbeta on Cys-179. J Biol Chem. 2006;281:35764–9.
51. Pergola PE, et al. Bardoxolone methyl and kidney function in CKD with type 2 diabetes. N Engl J Med. 2011;365:327–36.
52. de Zeeuw D, et al. Bardoxolone methyl in type 2 diabetes and stage 4 chronic kidney disease. N Engl J Med. 2013;369:2492–503.
53. Bakris GL, et al. Effect of finerenone on albuminuria in patients with diabetic nephropathy: a randomized clinical trial. JAMA. 2015;314:884–94.
54. Ito S, et al. Efficacy and safety of esaxerenone (CS-3150) for the treatment of type 2 diabetes with microalbuminuria: a randomized, double-blind, placebo-controlled, phase II trial. Clin J Am Soc Nephrol. 2019;14:1161–72.

Chapter 7
Nutrition and Diet Therapy for DKD

Shinji Kume

7.1 Introduction

Comprehensive therapy focusing on managing blood glucose levels, blood pressure, and the lipid profile is the most recommended therapeutic approach for diabetic kidney disease (DKD). This therapy aims to manage progression toward end-stage kidney disease and cardiovascular disease. Comprehensive therapy involves various approaches, such as improving lifestyle habits (diet and exercise therapies) and pharmacotherapy. Therefore, sharing of information and collaboration within a medical team, including a physician, nursing staff, and nutritionist, in planning and performing treatment and education of patients, are important for promoting better clinical outcomes in DKD. Among these approaches, diet therapy is an essential part of comprehensive therapy, and it needs to be tailored to suit the stage of DKD. In diet therapy, there are no clear guidelines on protein restriction, which is important because it depends on factors, such as age, nutritional status, adherence, and risk of cardiovascular disease. In this section, we outline some salient points and issues of diet therapy according to the stages of DKD and discuss remaining issues in diet therapy in DKD.

7.2 Diet Therapy for DKD

An overview of diet therapy for DKD is shown in Table 7.1. This overview was modified from a clinical guideline published from the Japan Diabetes Society. A limitation is that standardizing dietary therapy worldwide is difficult because the cause of diabetes is slightly different among countries. In the United States, the main cause of diabetes is severe insulin resistance due to obesity and relatively

S. Kume (✉)
Department of Medicine, Shiga University of Medical Science, Otsu, Shiga, Japan
e-mail: skume@belle.shiga-med.ac.jp

T. Wada et al. (eds.), *Diabetic Kidney Disease*,
https://doi.org/10.1007/978-981-15-9301-7_7

Table 7.1 Nutritional considerations for patients with diabetic kidney disease (DKD) based on the clinical guideline provided from the Japan Diabetes Society

DKD stage	Total energy (kcal/IBW kg/day)	Protein	Salt	Potassium
No albuminuria (<30 mg/gCre)	25–30	<20% (% of total calorie)	<6.0 (g/day) Individualized restriction if hypertension presents	Not restricted
Microalbuminuria (30–300 mg/gCre)	25–30	<20% (% of total calorie)	<6.0 (g/day) Individualized restriction if hypertension presents	Not restricted
Macroalbuminuria (30–300 mg/gCre) (eGFR≧45 ml/min/1.73 m^2)	25–30	0.8–1.0 (g/IBW kg/day)	<6.0 (g/day)	<2000 (mg/day) Individualized restriction if hyperkalemia presents
Macroalbuminuria (30–300 mg/gCre) (30 ≦ eGFR < 45 ml/min/1.73 m^2)	25–35	0.6–0.8 (g/IBW kg/day)	<6.0 (g/day)	<2000 (mg/day) Individualized restriction if hyperkalemia presents
Renal failure (eGFR ≦ 30)	25–35	0.6–0.8 (g/IBW kg/day)	<6.0 (g/day)	<1500 (mg/day) Individualized restriction if hyperkalemia presents

Cre creatinine, *eGFR* estimated glomerular filtration rate, *IBW* ideal body weight

insufficient insulin secretion. However, in some Asian countries including Japan, the cause of diabetes is commonly due to insufficient insulin secretion in addition to mild insulin resistance. Therefore, the dietary amount of each nutrient should be optimized and modified according to the health problem and situation in the individual country. Additionally, if available, diet therapy should be conducted according to a clinical guideline supplied in each country [1].

7.2.1 *Diet Therapy in Chronic Kidney Disease Stages G1A1-2 and G2A1-2*

7.2.1.1 Caloric Intake

The recommended caloric intake, taking into account the degree of obesity and degree of activity, is 25–30 kcal/ideal body weight (IBW) kg/day with a goal of a body mass index (BMI) <25 kg/m^2. Several studies have reported that decreasing the caloric intake in patients with diabetes and obesity results in decreased albuminuria, as well as improved control of blood glucose levels [2, 3]. Therefore, in patients with severe obesity, the caloric intake can be decreased to 20–25 kcal/IBW kg/day.

7.2.1.2 Protein Intake

Protein intake depends on people's habits in various countries. The diet of a person with diabetes should ideally comprise 50–60% carbohydrates, with 1–1.2 g of protein/kg of IBW per day, and lipids should comprise the rest of the diet. An excessive protein consumption of >1.3 g/IBW kg/day should be avoided for preventing initiation and progression of DKD.

However, when the proportion of energy from carbohydrates is 50–60% of the total energy, the quantity of proteins is generally 15–20%. Consequently, based on the total energy intake, protein intake is 1–1.5 g/IBW kg/day and can become greater than 1.3 g/IBW kg/day (Fig. 7.1). In particular, when the proportion of carbohydrates is 50–55%, provided that the proportion of lipids is less than 30%, the proportion of protein will increase, as well as intake of protein (Fig. 7.1). This situation raises the question of whether a high protein intake is harmful. A high protein intake might damage organs, including the kidneys. Halbesma et al. reported the possibility of an increased incidence of cardiovascular events in a group with high protein intake (1.38–3.27 g/kg/day) compared with a group with protein consumption of 1.10–1.26 g/kg/day [4]. The risk of kidney damage in healthy older subjects secondary to a high protein intake of 2.0 g/kg/day has been reported previously [5]. A long-term study over 11 years reported that in women with a slightly decreased

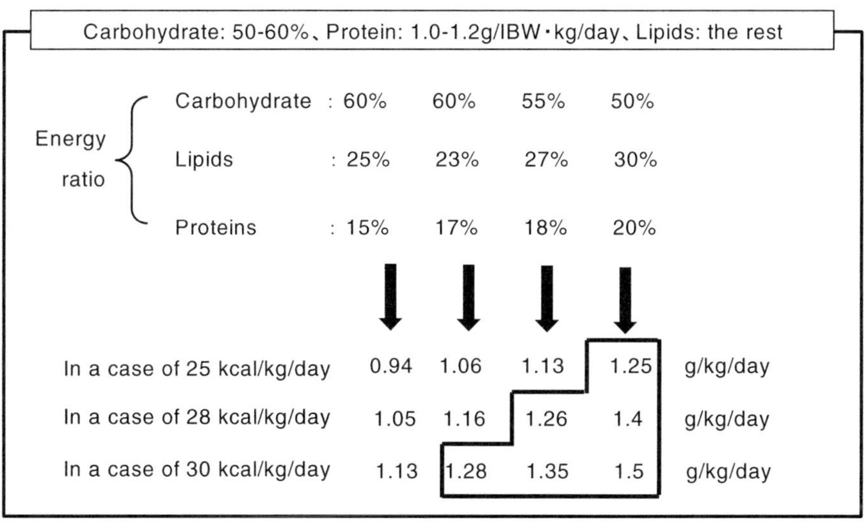

Fig. 7.1 The amount of protein intake in diet therapy for diabetic patients. Recommended protein intake in dietary therapy for diabetic patients is 15–20% of total energy or 1.0–1.5 g/IBW kg/day

renal function (estimated glomerular filtration rate [eGFR] of 55–88 ml/min/1.73 m^2), protein intake of >1.3 g/kg/day was associated with a progressive decrease in renal function (10 g/day increase in protein intake was associated with a decrease in eGFR of 7.72 ml/min/1.73 m^2) [5]. Therefore, even at this stage of DKD, when there is no clearly noticeable decrease in renal function, excessive protein intake of >1.3 g/IBW kg/day should be avoided because of the high risk of developing or worsening DKD and the risk of developing cardiovascular events.

Therefore, when prescribing low-carbohydrate diet therapy to decrease intake or improve blood glucose levels at this stage of DKD, restricting carbohydrates to less than 50% of the energy requirement should be avoided because of the risks associated with excess protein intake. An increase in protein intake should also be considered when prescribing diet therapy with a carbohydrate intake of 50–55%, and patients should be closely monitored in the long term.

7.2.1.3 Salt Restriction

Hypertension is a major concomitant disorder in diabetic patients. Especially, masked hypertension is a common feature in type 2 diabetic patients being treated for hypertension, and high sodium intake is associated with this type of hypertension [6]. In case of hypertension, regardless of causes, salt intake should be less than 6 g/day. Salt restriction is recommended because it has an independent depressor effect. When salt restriction is combined with medications, along with the depressor effect, an effect on improving proteinuria and renal function decline can be observed [7, 8]. However, excessive restriction of salt intake lowers appetite (especially in older subjects) and can also cause a deterioration in renal function secondary to dehydration. Therefore, careful monitoring is necessary in this situation. Additionally, there are varying views regarding the association between salt restriction and long-term prognosis or cardiovascular events [9]. Future prospective, long-term, intervention studies can help establish guidelines for this issue. In the diagnosis and treatment guide of chronic kidney disease (CKD) of 2012, which was provided by the Japanese Society of Nephrology, a daily salt intake of at least 3 or <6 g is recommended in cases of CKD, including DKD.

7.2.1.4 Potassium Intake

A high potassium intake, especially potassium citrate, stimulates sodium excretion into urine, leading to better blood pressure control. A recent observational study showed that higher urinary potassium excretion, which might reflect the daily potassium intake, was associated with the slower decline of renal function and the lower incidence of cardiovascular complications in type 2 diabetic patients with normal renal function [10]. Therefore, as long as patients do not have hyperkalemia or take a renin–angiotensin system inhibitor that elevates serum potassium levels as an adverse effect, potassium intake from fresh vegetables or fruits is recommended. To conclude the effectiveness of high potassium intake on DKD, interventional trials are necessary.

7.2.2 *Diet Therapy in CKD Stages G1-2A3 and G3-4*

In addition to the issue regarding calorie intake, the requirement for and practice of protein restriction from the macroalbuminuria stage onward is discussed in this section.

7.2.2.1 Caloric Intake

In the macroalbuminuria stage with an eGFR ≧ 45 ml/min/1.73 m^2 (CKD stage G1-2A3), the recommended caloric intake is 25–30 kcal/IBW kg/day (or 25–35 kcal/IBW kg/day depending on the degree of protein restriction) depending on the degree of obesity and degree of activity, with a goal of maintaining a BMI < 25 kg/m^2. In the patients with an eGFR < 45 ml/min/1.73 m^2, the recommended caloric intake is 25–35 kcal/IBW kg/day.

7.2.2.2 Restriction of Protein Intake

At present, protein restriction of 0.8–1.0 g/IBW kg/day should be performed from the stage of macroalbuminuria in DKD. Additionally, protein restriction to 0.6–0.8 g/IBW kg/day should be performed during the stage of renal dysfunction. Notably, protein restriction to 0.6–0.8 g/IBW kg/day should be considered even at the stage of macroalbuminuria from a GFR < 45 ml/min/1.73 m^2.

Protein restriction has been recommended because it is expected to improve glomerular hypertension/hyperfiltration and control progression of DKD by reducing the phosphorus and acid loads and reduce uremic toxicity and the need for dialysis. However, meta-analyses, systematic reviews, and randomized, controlled trials regarding the renoprotective effects of protein restriction in patients with DKD have shown controversial results [11–14]. Currently, evidence on this issue is unclear.

Consequently, various guidelines from countries, including the current American Diabetes Association guidelines, do not positively recommend protein restriction as diet therapy for DKD. Some of the reasons for unclear results regarding the renoprotective effect of protein restriction probably include problems with adherence to protein-restricted food, and the problem of which protein intake shows a renoprotective effect. A randomized, controlled trial with a duration of 5 years was carried out in Japan to determine the renoprotective effect of protein restriction in patients with type 2 diabetes with macroalbuminuria [12]. This trial did not show any obvious renoprotective effect of protein restriction [12]. This study also highlighted the difficulty of maintaining protein restriction over a long time. However, Nezu et al. reported the results of their meta-analysis, which indicated that GFR can be improved if protein restriction can be maintained [13]. Therefore, protein restriction can be expected to result in a consistent effect if it can be sustained. Consequently, renoprotective effects can be expected if there is clear adherence to the currently recommended protein restriction of 0.6–0.8 g/IBW kg/day. To achieve this goal, collaboration within a medical team is required.

Various researchers have investigated whether 0.6–0.8 g/IBW kg/day protein restriction is sufficient to demonstrate a renoprotective effect. Ideura et al. reported that in a clinical study on patients with glomerular nephritis (serum creatinine levels ≥6 mg/dL), a renoprotective effect was not observed with 0.6 g/IBW kg/day with protein restriction, but was observed with a higher degree of protein restriction (<0.5 g/IBW kg/day) [15]. Furthermore, Shimai et al. evaluated diabetic patients with severe renal dysfunction with serum creatinine levels ≥3.0 mg/dL and reported that a protein-restricted diet with 0.5 g/IBW kg/day resulted in a decrease in urine protein and delayed the need for dialysis treatment. However, these effects were not observed with a protein intake of ≥0.6 g/IBW kg/day. These results suggest that a more efficacious degree of protein restriction needs to be established to produce its renoprotective effects. Carrying out a high degree of protein restriction under current conditions in anticipation of renoprotective effects should be performed by using special low-protein food, with detailed physical evaluations by an experienced physician and nutritionist. This should be performed to avoid nutritional deficiencies such as those described below.

Protein restriction can be expected to have a consistent effect in protecting the kidneys, but more studies are required to establish the final guidelines. Furthermore, the quantity of protein required differs according to the age of an individual and individual nutritional status. Therefore, there is no single universal recommendation, and protein restriction should only be implemented after comprehensive evaluation of factors, such as age, pathology, risk, and compliance.

7.2.2.3 Issues of Performing Protein Restriction

After protein restriction is initiated, the nutritional status of the patient, including sarcopenia and frailty, as well as the course of proteinuria and renal function, should be evaluated. Although there are differences between reports on this issue depending on the method used to diagnose or evaluate nutritional disorders and the stage of CKD, protein–energy malnutrition (PEM) is found in approximately 20–50% of patients with CKD [16, 17]. Moreover, this state of malnutrition occurs during treatment prior to dialysis and the stage of dialysis and can contribute to an increased risk of cardiovascular disease and associated mortality rates via physical factors, such as chronic inflammation or increased oxidative stress. If adequate energy intake cannot be ensured when carrying out protein restriction, the protein consumed may not be efficiently used for protein synthesis, thus resulting in

PEM. Therefore, when performing protein restriction from the stage of severe kidney dysfunction, an energy intake of at least 30–35 kcal per kg of ideal or actual body weight (when BMI is <18.5 kg/m^2) is necessary. Additionally, 25 kcal per kg of ideal or actual body weight is possible in cases of obese subjects even before the stage of dialysis. Although increasing the intake of carbohydrate to ensure adequate energy intake during protein restriction is possible, this may lead to poorer control of blood glucose levels. Therefore, careful monitoring is necessary.

7.2.2.4 Restriction of Salt Intake

From this stage onward, salt restriction to 6 g/day is recommended, irrespective of the presence of concurrent hypertension. Salt restriction is especially recommended for patients with edema due to nephrotic-range proteinuria or cardiac dysfunction because uncontrollable fluid accumulation leads to early induction of dialysis therapy. However, as in the case of pre-DKD to microalbuminuria stages, careful monitoring is required to identify dehydration and a decrease in renal function due to excessive restriction of salt intake (especially when combined with renin–angiotensin system inhibitors and diuretics).

7.2.2.5 Potassium Restriction

Because many patients in this stage of DKD will be on renin–angiotensin system inhibitors for the expected renoprotective effect of these drugs, serum potassium levels should be monitored along with blood pressure. While potassium restriction is usually not necessary for all patients in the stage of macroalbuminuria, in the event of concurrent hyperkalemia, potassium should be restricted to <2 g/day, with restriction to <1.5 g/day in the stage of renal failure. Serum potassium levels should be managed within the range of 4.0–5.4 mEq/L.

7.2.2.6 Phosphorus Restriction

An elevation in serum phosphorus levels is thought to be strongly associated with CKD–mineral and bone disorder and secondary hyperparathyroidism in chronic renal failure and with ectopic calcification, including calcification of blood vessels. Additionally, a meta-analysis showed that elevation of serum phosphorus levels in patients with CKD is an independent risk factor for progression toward renal failure and an increased mortality rate [18]. Therefore, management of serum phosphorus levels is critically important to extend a healthy life span in patients with DKD.

Consequently, serum phosphorus should be maintained within the normal range (approximately 2.5–4.5 mg/dL) until initiation of renal replacement therapy. Additionally, phosphorus restriction should be included in diet therapy to avoid elevated serum phosphorus levels in the stage of renal failure when there is concurrent hyperphosphatemia. However, because there is an association of elevated serum phosphorus levels with protein intake, phosphorus restriction should be introduced in association with protein restriction. Phosphorus is present in cellular components, and therefore, nearly all foods contain phosphorus. Approximately all of the phosphorus is bound to proteins. Consequently, excess protein intake leads to an increased intake of phosphorus. However, in particular, foods with a high phosphorus/protein ratio, such as some dairy products, liver, small fish such as dried whitebait and shishamo smelt (*Spirinchus lanceolatus*), and other dried whole fish, should be avoided. Although phosphorus in food is organic phosphorus, many food additives include inorganic phosphorus. While only approximately half of the organic phosphorus ingested is absorbed, approximately 90% of inorganic phosphorus consumed is absorbed. Therefore, excessive consumption of fast foods, instant foods, soft drinks, snacks, and confectioneries, which contain a large amount of food additives, should be avoided to prevent excess ingestion of inorganic phosphorus and the resulting accumulation of phosphorus.

7.2.3 Other Issues in Diet Therapy of Clinical DKD

Quality control of each nutrient should be performed. Over the decades, many clinical studies have been conducted to identify the optimal amount of nutrients to prevent DKD. However, carbohydrates, proteins, and lipids include several types of nutrients in each of them. In foods, glucose and fructose are mainly contained. Fructose has been focused on as a poor food for DKD [19]. High level of serum uric acid is associated with progression of DKD and cardiovascular events in diabetic patients [20, 21]. High fructose intake stimulates uric acid production, resulting in progression of DKD [19, 22]. In a study, consumption of fructose-containing beverages representing 25% of energy requirements for 10 weeks significantly raised serum uric acid level, compared with the glucose-containing beverages [23]. In the National Health and Nutrition Examination Survey (NHANES), the consumption of sugar-sweetened soft drinks was positively associated with serum uric acid levels, suggesting that the fructose in soft drinks could increase uric acid levels [24]. Because soft drinks contain fructose as well as much inorganic phosphorus, for diabetic patients these sugar-sweetened soft drinks should not be recommended.

Dietary fatty acids consist of saturated and unsaturated fatty acids. Many clinical guidelines suggest that saturated fatty acids should be avoided, but unsaturated fatty acids, particularly omega-3 polyunsaturated fatty acid, are recommended for preventing vascular complications in diabetes [25].

Furthermore, some recent reports, including the Dietary Approaches to Stop Hypertension (DASH) Trial, have shown that a high intake of plant-based proteins has a benefit for controlling blood pressure and preventing CKD progression [26]. However, animal-based proteins are associated with progression of CKD [27, 28]. Collectively, we need to identify an optimal dietary therapy in DKD that is based on quality control of each nutrient, as well as quantity controls.

Hypoglycemia must be avoided, especially in patients who are treated with an insulin analog or oral agents that stimulate insulin secretion independently to blood glucose levels. Symptomatic hypoglycemia is associated with a higher mortality risk [29]. In diabetic patients with renal dysfunction, a hypoglycemic event frequently occurs, which must be prevented. Excess fluid intake also must be avoided for patients who have cardiac failure, renal failure, or nephrotic syndrome. Therefore, fasting carbohydrates that are suitable for patients with renal impairment include dextrose tablets, hard candy, honey, and non-cola regular pop instead of the generally recommended strategy with juice or cola beverages.

Increased proteinuria is a critical prognostic factor for developing CKD, regardless of kidney disease. Most diabetic patients with a CKD stage below G3 showed macroalbuminuria in the 1900s [30]. In contrast, recently, but the number of diabetic patients who have albuminuria has been decreasing, but the number of diabetic patients with a lower eGFR (<60 ml/min/1.73 m^2), even without albuminuria, has been increasing [30]. Currently, there is no clinical evidence of diet therapy for diabetic patients who have an early decline in the eGFR. In the future, an optimal dietary strategy for these patients should be provided.

7.2.4 Mechanisms Behind Dietary Therapy-Related Renoprotection in Experimental Diabetic Kidney Disease and Vascular Damage

Glomerular hypertension related to hyperactivation of the renin–angiotensin system (RAS) and intra- and extracellular metabolic alterations due to hyperglycemia and dyslipidemia are considered typical and classical aspects of the pathogenesis of DKD. Both of these factors lead to increased albuminuria and cell damage in a variety of cells including vascular endothelial cells, mesangial cells, podocytes, and tubular cells. These events synergistically injure the kidney, leading to progression of the stage of DKD.

Among dietary regimens, the mechanism behind protein restriction-mediated renoprotection has been the most extensively examined. Protein levels are linked to the activity of the RAS. Protein overload activates the RAS, whereas protein restriction suppresses the intrarenal RAS activation [31–33]. Peters et al. reported that RAS blockade and a low protein diet have additive effects on disease reduction in nephritic rats [34], suggesting that protein restriction exerts an additional mechanism to halt progression of kidney disease beyond RAS inhibitors. Furthermore, dietary protein overload increases the excretion of amino acids from the glomerulus, which leads to the increased reabsorption of amino acids, sodium, and chloride in the proximal tubules, resulting in a deficiency in the chloride levels achieved in the juxtaglomerular apparatus [35]. Subsequently, the tubular glomerular feedback system is activated. Then, the glomerular filtration rate is increased by protein overload [36]. Therefore, the modulation of intraglomerular pressure achieved with a protein restriction theoretically protects against the progression of DKD.

In addition to protein restriction, salt restriction also reduces hyperfiltration [37]. Thus, improvement of hemodynamic changes, particularly glomerular hyperfiltration, should be involved in the renoprotective mechanism of protein and salt restriction, possibly via reducing protein permeability of glomeruli.

Alterations of intra- and extracellular metabolism, such as oxidative stress, activation of PKC signaling, the polyol and hexosamine pathways, and excess accumulation of advanced glycated end products are classical ideas in DKD pathogenesis [38]. All these changes are due to hyperglycemia and dyslipidemia. Thus, amelioration of these pathogenic signals should be involved in the renoprotective mechanism of reducing calorie intake and resultant better body weight, glycemic, and lipid controls.

In addition to the traditional models of the pathogenesis of DKD, novel models of pathogenesis have been proposed experimentally. Vascular calcification is often observed in DKD patients and is associated with higher cardiovascular events and CKD progression [39]. Phosphorus metabolism is also strongly associated with these events. Experimentally, phosphorus toxicity caused vascular calcification-related endothelial dysfunction and CKD progression [40]. Thus, the restriction of dietary phosphorus should receive more attention to prevent vascular injury-related CVD events and DKD progression.

Intracellular nutrient sensing systems are currently being focused on as another promising model for the pathogenesis of DKD [41]. Nutrient-sensing signals and their related intracellular machinery have evolved to combat prolonged periods of starvation in mammals; and these systems are conserved in the kidney. Recent studies have suggested that the activity of three nutrient-sensing signals, mechanistic target of rapamycin complex 1 (mTORC1), AMP-activated protein kinase (AMPK) and mammalian homolog of sirtuin 1 (Sirt1), is altered in the diabetic kidney. In animal models of experimental DKD, hyperactivation of mTORC1 caused severe podocyte injury and obesity-related proximal tubular cell damage [42, 43]. A diabetes-related decrease in AMPK activity is also associated with DKD [44]. Furthermore, Sirt1 activity in proximal tubular cells and podocytes decreased in streptozotocin-induced diabetic mice, which was associated with increased proteinuria [45]. Interestingly, protein restriction suppressed mTORC1 signaling in diabetic kidneys of rats [46] and calorie restriction preserved both Sirt1 and AMPK activation [47]. Thus, normalization of all these signals may be involved in protein restriction- and calorie restriction-mediated renoprotection in DKD.

Furthermore, autophagy activity, which is regulated by the abovementioned nutrient-sensing signals, is also altered in both podocytes and proximal tubular cells under diabetic conditions [43, 48]. Under diabetic conditions, an altered nutritional state owing to nutrient excess may disturb cellular homeostasis regulated by nutrient-sensitive systems, leading to exacerbation of organelle dysfunction and DKD. Interestingly, in diabetic rats, decreased autophagy activity in diabetes was reversed upon protein restriction, which resulted in maintenance of normal mitochondrial morphology and function [46]. Interestingly, excess phosphorus is also likely to weaken autophagy activity. Thus, reactivation of autophagy may play a central role in renoprotection due to protein restriction, calorie restriction, and phosphorus restriction in DKD.

7.3 Conclusion

This section outlined diet therapy in DKD according to the stages of this disease from the pre-DKD stage to the stage of renal failure. Important questions to consider regarding diet therapy in DKD in the pre-dialysis stages are whether protein restriction should be implemented, and if it should, at what stage and to what degree? However, there are numerous issues that remain to be studied, such as the degree of protein restriction, quality of protein required (animal or plant), and the balance between amino acids to achieve a renoprotective effect.

In routine diagnosis and treatment, a diabetic diet based on energy restriction should be switched to a diet for DKD based on protein restriction with an adequate energy intake to prevent PEM. However, depending on the individual patient's characteristics, the results can be ambiguous. To avoid this situation, microalbuminuria needs to be correctly diagnosed, and the patient should be educated from this stage of the disease to avoid future development toward renal failure. At any stage of DKD, the type of diet therapy should be tailored to each individual after considering age, compliance, and overall physical condition. Additionally, after introducing diet therapy, the efficacy of the diet needs to be evaluated by monitoring body weight, performing a nutritional evaluation, conducting a physical examination, and compliance over time.

References

1. Whitham D. Nutrition for the prevention and treatment of chronic kidney disease in diabetes. Can J Diabetes. 2014;38(5):344–8.
2. Look ARG, Pi-Sunyer X, Blackburn G, Brancati FL, Bray GA, Bright R, et al. Reduction in weight and cardiovascular disease risk factors in individuals with type 2 diabetes: one-year results of the look AHEAD trial. Diabetes Care. 2007;30(6):1374–83.
3. Morales E, Valero MA, Leon M, Hernandez E, Praga M. Beneficial effects of weight loss in overweight patients with chronic proteinuric nephropathies. Am J Kidney Dis. 2003;41(2):319–27.
4. Halbesma N, Bakker SJ, Jansen DF, Stolk RP, De Zeeuw D, De Jong PE, et al. High protein intake associates with cardiovascular events but not with loss of renal function. J Am Soc Nephrol. 2009;20(8):1797–804.
5. Walrand S, Short KR, Bigelow ML, Sweatt AJ, Hutson SM, Nair KS. Functional impact of high protein intake on healthy elderly people. Am J Physiol Endocrinol Metab. 2008;295(4):E921–8.
6. Uzu T, Nakao K, Kume S, Araki H, Isshiki K, Araki S, et al. High sodium intake is associated with masked hypertension in Japanese patients with type 2 diabetes and treated hypertension. Am J Hypertens. 2012;25(11):1170–4.

7. Kanauchi N, Ookawara S, Ito K, Mogi S, Yoshida I, Kakei M, et al. Factors affecting the progression of renal dysfunction and the importance of salt restriction in patients with type 2 diabetic kidney disease. Clin Exp Nephrol. 2015;19(6):1120–6.
8. Parvanova A, Trillini M, Podesta MA, Iliev IP, Ruggiero B, Abbate M, et al. Moderate salt restriction with or without paricalcitol in type 2 diabetes and losartan-resistant macroalbuminuria (PROCEED): a randomised, double-blind, placebo-controlled, crossover trial. Lancet Diabetes Endocrinol. 2018;6(1):27–40.
9. Taylor RS, Ashton KE, Moxham T, Hooper L, Ebrahim S. Reduced dietary salt for the prevention of cardiovascular disease: a meta-analysis of randomized controlled trials (Cochrane review). Am J Hypertens. 2011;24(8):843–53.
10. Araki S, Haneda M, Koya D, Kondo K, Tanaka S, Arima H, et al. Urinary potassium excretion and renal and cardiovascular complications in patients with type 2 diabetes and normal renal function. Clin J Am Soc Nephrol. 2015;10(12):2152–8.
11. Hansen HP, Tauber-Lassen E, Jensen BR, Parving HH. Effect of dietary protein restriction on prognosis in patients with diabetic nephropathy. Kidney Int. 2002;62(1):220–8.
12. Koya D, Haneda M, Inomata S, Suzuki Y, Suzuki D, Makino H, et al. Long-term effect of modification of dietary protein intake on the progression of diabetic nephropathy: a randomised controlled trial. Diabetologia. 2009;52(10):2037–45.
13. Nezu U, Kamiyama H, Kondo Y, Sakuma M, Morimoto T, Ueda S. Effect of low-protein diet on kidney function in diabetic nephropathy: meta-analysis of randomised controlled trials. BMJ Open. 2013;3(5):e002934.
14. Pan Y, Guo LL, Jin HM. Low-protein diet for diabetic nephropathy: a meta-analysis of randomized controlled trials. Am J Clin Nutr. 2008;88(3):660–6.
15. Ideura T, Shimazui M, Morita H, Yoshimura A. Protein intake of more than 0.5 g/kg BW/day is not effective in suppressing the progression of chronic renal failure. Contrib Nephrol. 2007;155:40–9.
16. Pupim LB, Cuppari L, Ikizler TA. Nutrition and metabolism in kidney disease. Semin Nephrol. 2006;26(2):134–57.
17. Stenvinkel P, Heimburger O, Paultre F, Diczfalusy U, Wang T, Berglund L, et al. Strong association between malnutrition, inflammation, and atherosclerosis in chronic renal failure. Kidney Int. 1999;55(5):1899–911.
18. Da J, Xie X, Wolf M, Disthabanchong S, Wang J, Zha Y, et al. Serum phosphorus and progression of CKD and mortality: a meta-analysis of cohort studies. Am J Kidney Dis. 2015;66(2):258–65.
19. Bjornstad P, Lanaspa MA, Ishimoto T, Kosugi T, Kume S, Jalal D, et al. Fructose and uric acid in diabetic nephropathy. Diabetologia. 2015;58(9):1993–2002.
20. Ficociello LH, Rosolowsky ET, Niewczas MA, Maselli NJ, Weinberg JM, Aschengrau A, et al. High-normal serum uric acid increases risk of early progressive renal function loss in type 1 diabetes: results of a 6-year follow-up. Diabetes Care. 2010;33(6):1337–43.
21. Jalal DI, Rivard CJ, Johnson RJ, Maahs DM, McFann K, Rewers M, et al. Serum uric acid levels predict the development of albuminuria over 6 years in patients with type 1 diabetes: findings from the Coronary Artery Calcification in Type 1 Diabetes study. Nephrol Dial Transplant. 2010;25(6):1865–9.
22. Stirpe F, Della Corte E, Bonetti E, Abbondanza A, Abbati A, De Stefano F. Fructose-induced hyperuricaemia. Lancet. 1970;2(7686):1310–1.
23. Cox CL, Stanhope KL, Schwarz JM, Graham JL, Hatcher B, Griffen SC, et al. Consumption of fructose- but not glucose-sweetened beverages for 10 weeks increases circulating concentrations of uric acid, retinol binding protein-4, and gamma-glutamyl transferase activity in overweight/obese humans. Nutr Metab (Lond). 2012;9(1):68.
24. Choi JW, Ford ES, Gao X, Choi HK. Sugar-sweetened soft drinks, diet soft drinks, and serum uric acid level: the Third National Health and Nutrition Examination Survey. Arthritis Rheum. 2008;59(1):109–16.

25. Shapiro H, Theilla M, Attal-Singer J, Singer P. Effects of polyunsaturated fatty acid consumption in diabetic nephropathy. Nat Rev Nephrol. 2011;7(2):110–21.
26. Rebholz CM, Crews DC, Grams ME, Steffen LM, Levey AS, Miller ER 3rd, et al. DASH (dietary approaches to stop hypertension) diet and risk of subsequent kidney disease. Am J Kidney Dis. 2016;68(6):853–61.
27. Haring B, Selvin E, Liang M, Coresh J, Grams ME, Petruski-Ivleva N, et al. dietary protein sources and risk for incident chronic kidney disease: results from the Atherosclerosis Risk in Communities (ARIC) study. J Ren Nutr. 2017;27(4):233–42.
28. Lew QJ, Jafar TH, Koh HW, Jin A, Chow KY, Yuan JM, et al. Red meat intake and risk of ESRD. J Am Soc Nephrol. 2017;28(1):304–12.
29. Ismail-Beigi F, Craven T, Banerji MA, Basile J, Calles J, Cohen RM, et al. Effect of intensive treatment of hyperglycaemia on microvascular outcomes in type 2 diabetes: an analysis of the ACCORD randomised trial. Lancet. 2010;376(9739):419–30.
30. Afkarian M, Zelnick LR, Hall YN, Heagerty PJ, Tuttle K, Weiss NS, et al. Clinical manifestations of kidney disease among US adults with diabetes, 1988–2014. JAMA. 2016;316(6):602–10.
31. Martinez-Maldonado M, Benabe JE, Wilcox JN, Wang S, Luo C. Renal renin, angiotensinogen, and ANG I-converting-enzyme gene expression: influence of dietary protein. Am J Phys. 1993;264(6 Pt 2):F981–8.
32. Benabe JE, Fernandez-Repollet E, Tapia E, Luo C, Martinez-Maldonado M. Angiotensin II and catecholamines interaction in short-term low protein feeding. Kidney Int. 1993;44(2):285–93.
33. Benabe JE, Wang S, Wilcox JN, Martinez-Maldonado M. Modulation of ANG II receptor and its mRNA in normal rat by low-protein feeding. Am J Phys. 1993;265(5 Pt 2):F660–9.
34. Peters H, Border WA, Noble NA. Angiotensin II blockade and low-protein diet produce additive therapeutic effects in experimental glomerulonephritis. Kidney Int. 2000;57(4):1493–501.
35. Gonska T, Hirsch JR, Schlatter E. Amino acid transport in the renal proximal tubule. Amino Acids. 2000;19(2):395–407.
36. Sallstrom J, Carlstrom M, Olerud J, Fredholm BB, Kouzmine M, Sandler S, et al. High-protein-induced glomerular hyperfiltration is independent of the tubuloglomerular feedback mechanism and nitric oxide synthases. Am J Physiol Regul Integr Comp Physiol. 2010;299(5):R1263–8.
37. Lau C, Sudbury I, Thomson M, Howard PL, Magil AB, Cupples WA. Salt-resistant blood pressure and salt-sensitive renal autoregulation in chronic streptozotocin diabetes. Am J Physiol Regul Integr Comp Physiol. 2009;296(6):R1761–70.
38. Brownlee M. The pathobiology of diabetic complications: a unifying mechanism. Diabetes. 2005;54(6):1615–25.
39. Sigrist MK, Taal MW, Bungay P, McIntyre CW. Progressive vascular calcification over 2 years is associated with arterial stiffening and increased mortality in patients with stages 4 and 5 chronic kidney disease. Clin J Am Soc Nephrol. 2007;2(6):1241–8.
40. Scialla JJ, Lau WL, Reilly MP, Isakova T, Yang HY, Crouthamel MH, et al. Fibroblast growth factor 23 is not associated with and does not induce arterial calcification. Kidney Int. 2013;83(6):1159–68.
41. Kume S, Thomas MC, Koya D. Nutrient sensing, autophagy, and diabetic nephropathy. Diabetes. 2012;61(1):23–9.
42. Inoki K, Mori H, Wang J, Suzuki T, Hong S, Yoshida S, et al. mTORC1 activation in podocytes is a critical step in the development of diabetic nephropathy in mice. J Clin Invest. 2011;121(6):2181–96.
43. Yamahara K, Kume S, Koya D, Tanaka Y, Morita Y, Chin-Kanasaki M, et al. Obesity-mediated autophagy insufficiency exacerbates proteinuria-induced tubulointerstitial lesions. J Am Soc Nephrol. 2013;24(11):1769–81.
44. Zhao J, Miyamoto S, You YH, Sharma K. AMP-activated protein kinase (AMPK) activation inhibits nuclear translocation of Smad4 in mesangial cells and diabetic kidneys. Am J Physiol Renal Physiol. 2015;308(10):F1167–77.

45. Hasegawa K, Wakino S, Simic P, Sakamaki Y, Minakuchi H, Fujimura K, et al. Renal tubular Sirt1 attenuates diabetic albuminuria by epigenetically suppressing Claudin-1 overexpression in podocytes. Nat Med. 2013;19(11):1496–504.
46. Kitada M, Ogura Y, Suzuki T, Sen S, Lee SM, Kanasaki K, et al. A very-low-protein diet ameliorates advanced diabetic nephropathy through autophagy induction by suppression of the mTORC1 pathway in Wistar fatty rats, an animal model of type 2 diabetes and obesity. Diabetologia. 2016;59(6):1307–17.
47. Kume S, Uzu T, Horiike K, Chin-Kanasaki M, Isshiki K, Araki S, et al. Calorie restriction enhances cell adaptation to hypoxia through Sirt1-dependent mitochondrial autophagy in mouse aged kidney. J Clin Invest. 2010;120(4):1043–55.
48. Tagawa A, Yasuda M, Kume S, Yamahara K, Nakazawa J, Chin-Kanasaki M, et al. Impaired podocyte autophagy exacerbates proteinuria in diabetic nephropathy. Diabetes. 2016;65(3):755–67.

Chapter 8
Renal Structural-Functional Relationships at the Early Stage of Diabetic Nephropathy Among Types 1 and 2 Diabetes: Similarity and Difference

Tatsumi Moriya

8.1 Renal Histological Changes and Clinical Manifestations of Diabetic Nephropathy in Type 1 and Type 2 Diabetes

In types 1 and 2 diabetes, the clinical manifestations of diabetic nephropathy include an increase in albuminuria or a decline in the renal function. Once clinical findings, i.e., macroalbuminuria, are apparently manifest, there are already severe histological changes and renal function decline often progresses. Therefore, we need to confirm early renal structural-functional relationships before clinical parameters become obvious.

8.2 Renal Pathological Findings in Types 1 and 2 Patients

8.2.1 Typical Renal Histological Findings as Diabetic Glomerulosclerosis

Typical pathological findings are glomerular basement membrane (GBM) thickening, mesangial expansion, tubular atrophy, tubulointersitial expansion or fibrosis, and arteriolar hyalinosis in both types 1 and 2 diabetes (Figs. 8.1a, b and 8.2). These changes are well known both in types 1 and 2 diabetic patients with macroalbuminuria; however, we can see some of these histological changes even in diabetic patients at the normoalbuminuric stage (Table 8.1). Although a persistent increase

T. Moriya (✉)
Health Care Center, Kitasato University, Sagamihara, Kanagawa, Japan
e-mail: moriy@kitasato-u.ac.jp

T. Wada et al. (eds.), *Diabetic Kidney Disease*,
https://doi.org/10.1007/978-981-15-9301-7_8

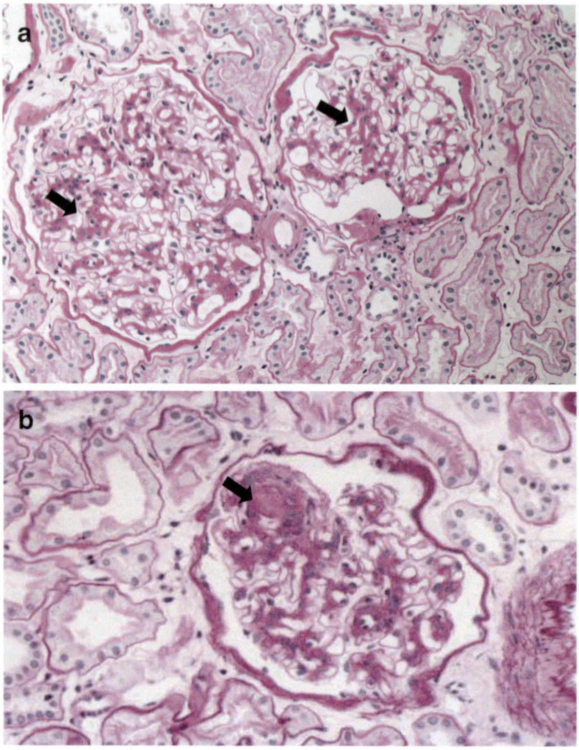

Fig. 8.1 Light microscopic micrographs show that mesangial expansion (**a**; arrows) and nodular glomerulosclerosis (**b**; arrow) can be seen in normoalbuminuric diabetic patients (PAS stain)

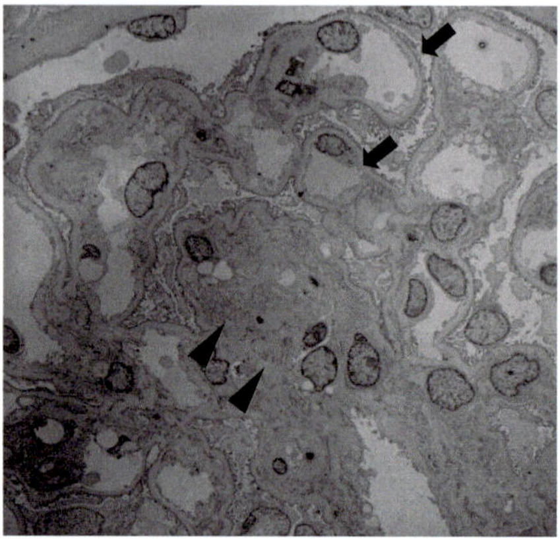

Fig. 8.2 Electron microscopic micrograph shows a part of glomerulus in normoalbuminuric type 2 diabetic patients. GBM thickening (arrows) and mesangial expansion (arrowheads) have already been present in this case

in the levels of urinary albumin excretion in the microalbuminuria range is currently the best early biomarker for the risk of diabetic nephropathy, histological lesions in types 1 and 2 diabetes may be quite advanced before microalbuminuria develops [1, 2].

Table 8.1 Histological findings of diabetic nephropathy

1. Glomerular change
GBM thickening[a]
Mesangial expansion[a]
Diffuse lesion
Nodular lesion
Podocyte loss and foot process width enlargement
Decrease in endothelial fenestration[a]
2. Tubulointerstitial change
TBM thickening[a]
Interstitial expansion or fibrosis[a]
3. Vascular change
Arteriolar hyalinosis[a]
Atherosclerosis
Neovascularization at the vascular pore
4. Changes in JGA
JGA enlargement[a]
T cell infiltration to the JGA[a]
5. Others

JGA juxtaglomerular apparatus
[a]Can be seen in normoalbuminuric stage

8.2.2 Morphometric Analysis of Renal Biopsies

Stereological morphometry should be performed to evaluate quantitatively renal structural changes using both light and electron microscopic materials. It is very important to obtain the systematic unbiased and efficient number of samples from the reference areas in the materials. It is suggested to refer the previous papers [3–6] regarding the detail of morphometric analysis. Brief description regarding methodology of morphometric analysis in our institute is described as below.

8.2.2.1 Light Microscopic (LM) Morphometric Analysis

Renal biopsy tissue was fixed in 10% buffered formalin and stained with periodic acid-Schiff stain. The mean glomerular volume (MGV) was determined from the LM sections at an approximate magnification of ×150 using the point counting method of Weibel and Gomez [7]. Percent global glomerular sclerosis (%GS) was measured as described previously [8]. At least 15 glomerular profiles for each patient were measured for MGV and %GS. Interstitial volume fraction [Vv(Int/cortex)] was determined from the LM sections at an approximate magnification of ×300 by point-counting images projected onto a white surface using a projection microscope [4]. The index of arteriolar hyalinosis (IAH) score was obtained by the estimation of the fraction of each arteriolar wall replaced by hyaline in one complete LM section [9, 10].

In addition, the renal injury patterns of the LM tissues are categorized according to the previous study by Fioretto et al. [11]:

- Category I (CI): normal or near normal renal structure. These patients had biopsies that were normal or showed very mild mesangial expansion, tubulointerstitial changes, or arteriolar hyalinosis in any combination.
- Category II (CII): typical diabetic glomerulopathy with parallel changes in the tubulointerstitium and vessels. These patients had established diabetic lesions with balanced severity of glomerular, tubulointerstitial, and arteriolar changes.
- Category III (CIII): atypical injury patterns, absent or mild diabetic glomerulopathy associated with disproportionately severe tubulointerstitial injury, and/or arteriolar hyalinosis, and/or global glomerular sclerosis.

8.2.2.2 Electron Microscopic (EM) Morphometry

All specimens were cut into thick and 80–90 nm ultrathin sections and studied using a JEOL CX 100 transmission electron microscope (JEOL, Tokyo, Japan) in the Kitasato Bio-Imaging Center. Kidney tissues were cut into 1 mm^3 cubes, fixed in 2.5% glutaraldehyde in 0.2 M cacodylate buffer (pH 7.4), and post-fixed in osmium tetroxide. These specimens were dehydrated in a graded ethanol series and embedded in Quetol 812 (Nissin EM Inc., Tokyo, Japan). All specimens were cut into thick and 80–90 nm ultrathin sections. At least two and usually three non-sclerosed glomeruli per biopsy were measured. The centermost glomerulus from each block was selected. Globally sclerosed glomeruli were excluded. Routine stereologic techniques, which have been previously described [3, 5, 6, 12], were used to measure the GBM width, mesangial fractional volume [Vv(Mes/glom)], and the surface density of the peripheral GBM [Sv(PGBM/glom)]. Briefly, the GBM width was measured using the orthogonal intercept method [5], Vv(Mes/glom) was measured by point counting, and Sv(PGBM/glom) was measured using the line-intercept method [3, 6, 12]. The number of measurements performed in each biopsy to estimate GBM width was usually over 100.

8.3 Renal Structural-Functional Relationships at the Early Stage of Diabetic Nephropathy in Types 1 and 2 Diabetic Patients

8.3.1 Cross-Sectional Studies

8.3.1.1 Renal Structure and Albuminuria

Previous studies have shown that urinary albumin excretion increases in parallel with GBM thickening and mesangial expansion in patients with type 1 diabetes [6, 13]. Caramori et al. [14] showed that the severity of glomerular

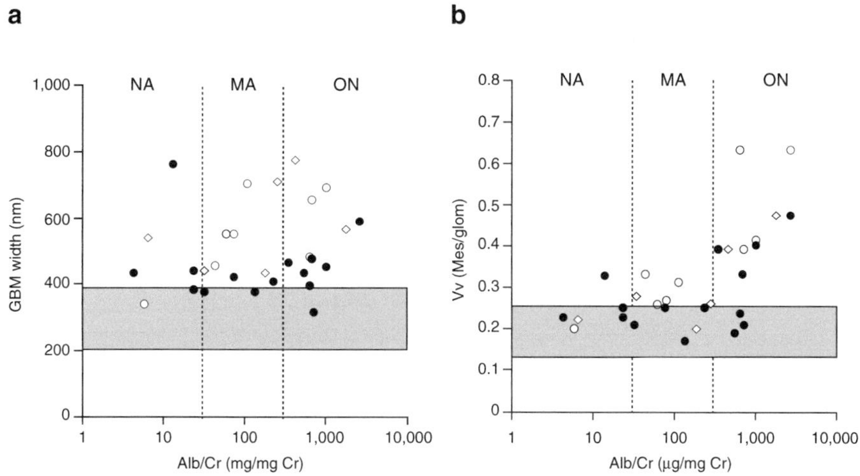

Fig. 8.3 (**a**) Individual values of GBM width among the three groups without retinopathy (closed circle) and with background (open circle) or preproliferative or proliferative (open diamond) retinopathy. The shaded area represents the mean ± 2 SD for GBM width in normal Japanese subjects. The dashed lines show the boundaries between normoalbuminuria (NA) and microalbuminuria (MA) and between MA and macroalbuminuria (ON). The GBM width overlapped completely among the three clinical categories. (**b**) Individual values of Vv(Mes/glom) among three groups without retinopathy (closed circle) and with background (open circle) or preproliferative or proliferative (open diamond) retinopathy. The shaded area represents the mean ± 2 SD for Vv(Mes/glom) in normal Japanese subjects. The dashed lines show the boundaries between NA and MA and between MA and ON. Vv(Mes/glom) overlapped completely among NA and MA patients, while the ON patients had higher Vv(Mes/glom) values than NA and MA patients

lesions, such as GBM thickening and mesangial expansion, increased significantly in patients with type 1 diabetes who had normo-, micro-, or macroalbuminuria. However, there was considerable overlap in these structural parameters between these categories of urinary albumin excretion. On the other hand, GBM thickness and mesangial expanded degree are not different between normoalbuminuria and microalbuminuria in type 2 diabetic patients [12] although these two histological parameters significantly increased in macroalbuminuric patients (Fig. 8.3a, b).

8.3.1.2 Renal Structure and Glomerular Filtration Rate (GFR)

The cross-sectional studies showed that the GFR was associated with the glomerular surface area in patients with types 1 and 2 diabetes [15–17] (Fig. 8.4). However, it is not fully elucidated that GFR decline occurred according to glomerular surface volume decreases during long time observation both in types 1 and 2 diabetes.

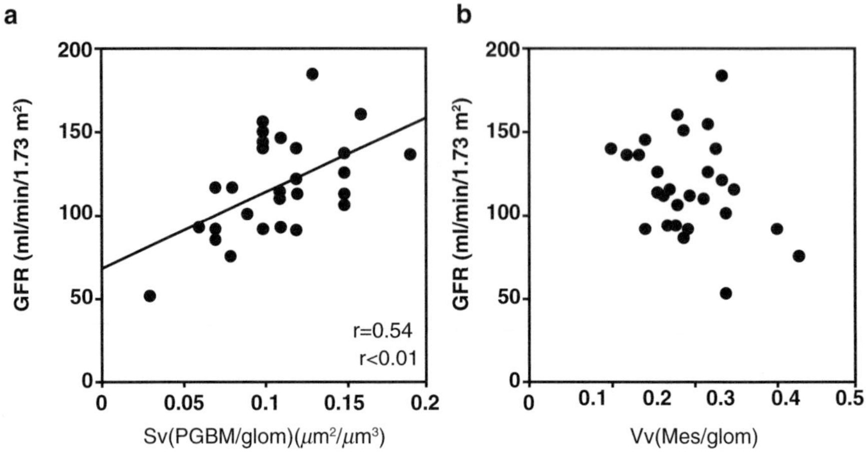

Fig. 8.4 The surface density of the peripheral glomerular basement membrane [Sv(PGBM/glom)] (**a**) and the volume fraction of the mesangium [Vv(Mes/glom)] (**b**) were compared with the baseline GFR data. The straight line in A indicates a statistically significant linear regression line (GFR = 449.2 × Sv(PGBM/glom) + 68.6, $r = 0.54$, $P < 0.01$)

8.3.2 *Longitudinal Studies*

8.3.2.1 Renal Histological Findings as Predictors for Renal Functional Decline in Types 1 and 2 Diabetic Patients

It is difficult to identify patients with type 2 diabetes who are at risk of developing progressive diabetic nephropathy because of a lack of sensitivity in the commonly used measurements of GFR and urinary albumin excretion. This has led to the exploration of renal histological changes as a measure of susceptibility to diabetic nephropathy. Various longitudinal studies have shown that histological parameters can be used to predict a decline in the renal function or an increase in albuminuria in patients with type 1 and 2 diabetes [14, 18]. In fact, it was shown that GBM thickening was a risk factor for the development of macroalbuminuria or end-stage kidney disease in normoalbuminuric patients with type 1 diabetes [14]. In Japanese patients with type 2 diabetes, GBM thickening and mesangial expansion predicted an increase in albuminuria after 6 years of follow-up [18]. Regarding the course of the renal function, in a study using research biopsies, GBM thickening and mesangial expansion were shown to predict a decline in the GFR in micro- and macroalbuminuric patients with type 2 diabetes [19] during 2.0–6.0 follow-up years. Moreover, several recent reports showed structural parameters indicating a loss of renal function in Pima Indian [20], Japanese [21, 22], and Chinese [23] patients with type 2 diabetes. However, most of the patients in these studies were macroalbuminuric.

8.3.2.2 Renal Histological Heterogeneity and Renal Functional Changes

Currently, there are insufficient longitudinal data to show which structural changes predict the slope of GFR decline in types 1 and 2 diabetic patients including those in the normoalbuminuric stage. Therefore, normotensive type 2 diabetic patients without macroalbuminuria, hematuria, or renal dysfunction and without any evidence suggesting atherosclerotic diseases were analyzed at the outpatient clinics of Akita, Nara, Niigata, and Kitasato University Hospitals in Japan in the previous study [24]. These renal tissues were divided into three histological categories according to the previous study [11]. Baseline and follow-up urinary albumin excretion were not different among the three groups. However, urinary albumin excretion was significantly increased in the CII group at the follow-up, and initial and final albuminuria stages were significantly different in the CII group. The eGFR among the groups did not differ at the baseline or the follow-up. However, the eGFRs in the CII and CIII patients were significantly decreased during the 11-year follow-up. The decrease of eGFR in the CI group was slightly greater than age-related renal function loss [25], which was under 1.0 ml/min/1.73 m^2 per year with no change between baseline and follow-up. Therefore, renal function in patients with normal or near normal renal structure remained unchanged, during this 11-year follow-up. However, the slope of eGFR decline was significantly greater among the CII patients than in the CI patients, while the urinary albumin excretion and the proportion of macroalbuminuria increased significantly in the CII patients at the follow-up (Table 8.2).

Table 8.2 Renal function at the initial and final stages and its change during the 11-year observation period

Characteristic	CI (n = 12)	CII (n = 14)	CIII (n = 11)	ANOVA
Initial eGFR (ml/min/1.73 m^2)	88.0 ± 14.9	93.9 ± 26.1	93.9 ± 17.2	NS
Final eGFR (ml/min/1.73 m^2)	76.5 ± 24.4	59.9 ± 21.5	76.6 ± 13.1	NS (0.07)
Slope of eGFR decline (ml/min/1.73 m^2/year)	−1.08 ± 1.23	−4.11 ± 3.99	−1.69 ± 1.96	0.02
P-value (initial vs. final eGFR)	NS	0.0001	0.0058	–
Initial ACR (mg/gCr)	25.9 (2.2–277.1)	50.9 (7.4–169.8)	15.8 (5.6–251.0)	NS
Final ACR (mg/gCr)	16.2 (0.2–1403.2)	162.8 (2.4–4135.9)	44.9 (3.1–367.2)	NS
P-value (initial vs. final ACR)	NS	<0.05	NS	–
Initial albuminuria stage (NA/MA/ON)	7/5/0	5/9/0	7/4/0	NS
Final albuminuria stage (NA/MA/ON)	7/3/2	4/4/6	5/5/1	NS
P-value (initial vs. final albuminuria stage)	NS	$P < 0.05$ (χ^2=8.0)	NS	–

8.3.2.3 Arteriolar Hyalinosis and Renal Functional Changes

Another LM finding, arteriolar hyalinosis, is not a specific histological finding in diabetic nephropathy (Fig. 8.5). However, it is a common finding and its severity can easily be estimated using LM. Moreover, the presence of both afferent and efferent glomerular arteriolar hyalinosis is virtually diagnostic of diabetic nephropathy. In our previous study, arteriolar hyalinosis was increased in patients with type 2 diabetes who were microalbuminuric compared to those with normoalbuminuria [24]. In type 1 diabetes, a cross-sectional study showed that arteriolar hyalinosis was related to global glomerular sclerosis and to both creatinine clearance and urinary albumin excretion [8]. However, there are no studies in the literature on the predictive value of arteriolar hyalinosis on the changes in GFR and urinary albumin excretion in type 2 diabetes. Although two recent reports investigated the relationship between renal structural parameters and renal functional loss in Pima Indians [20] and Japanese patients [21], the first report did not examine arteriolar hyalinosis [20], and the second report focused almost exclusively on macroalbuminuric patients [21]. Another study in Japanese patients with type 2 diabetes showed that arteriolar hyalinosis was associated with a low estimated GFR (eGFR), but, again, mainly focused on macroalbuminuric patients [22]. Renal survival was not related to arteriolar hyalinosis in Chinese patients with type 2 diabetes also mainly with macroalbuminuria [26].

In the previous study [10], Vv(Mes/glom) was negatively correlated with follow-up GFR ($r = -0.401$, $P = 0.033$) but did not correlate with UAE. On the other hand, the index of arteriolar hyalinosis (IAH) score was negatively correlated with GFR ($r = -0.491$, $P = 0.008$) (Fig. 8.6a) and positively correlated with UAE ($r = 0.420$, $P = 0.007$) (Fig. 8.6b) at follow-up. The IAH score was <2.0 in 22 patients and ≥2.0 in seven patients (Table 8.3). There were no significant differences in age, known duration of diabetes, HbA_{1c}, UAE at baseline, GFR at baseline, MGV,

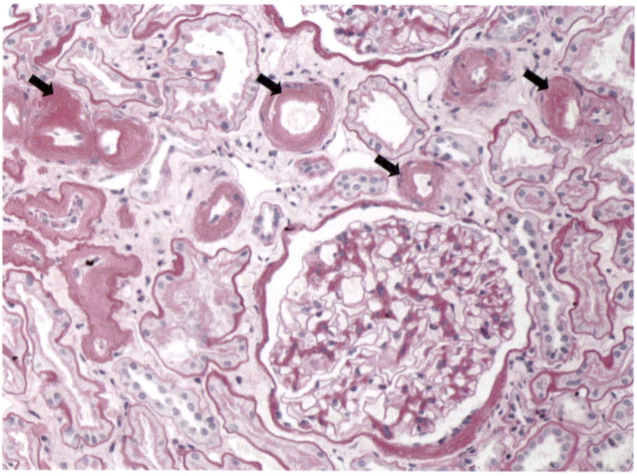

Fig. 8.5 Light microscopic findings show interstitial expansion and arteriolar hyalinosis (arrows) in normoalbuminuric type 2 diabetic patients

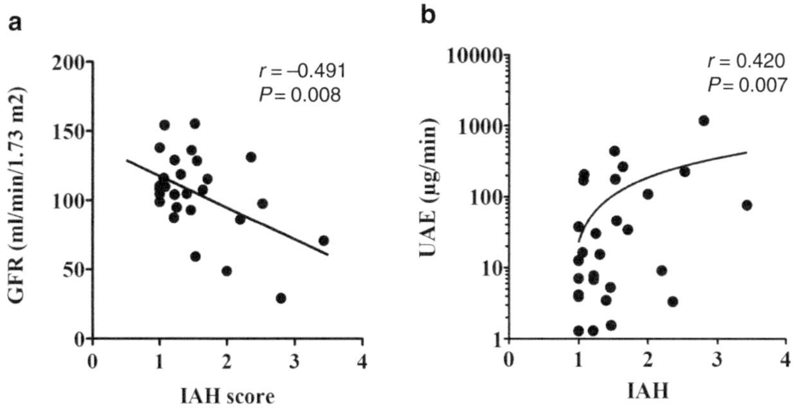

Fig. 8.6 The relationship of the index of arteriolar hyalinosis (IAH) score with glomerular filtration rate (GFR) (**a**) and urinary albumin excretion rate (UAE) (**b**) at follow-up. The IAH score was significantly and negatively correlated with GFR at the final observation ($r = -0.491$, $P = 0.008$). The IAH score was significantly and positively correlated with UAE at the final observation ($r = 0.420$, $P = 0.007$)

Vv(Int/cortex), %GS, GBM width, Vv(Mes/glom), or Sv(PGBM/glom) between patients with IAH scores <2.0 and ≥2.0. However, GFR at follow-up in patients with IAH scores ≥2.0 significantly decreased from baseline ($P = 0.025$) and was significantly lower than that of the patients with IAH scores <2.0 ($P = 0.005$), which did not decrease significantly from baseline (Table 8.3). The stepwise regression analysis showed that only the IAH score significantly affected GFR at the final observation ($F = 5.20$, $P = 0.036$) (Table 8.4). Other histological findings including mesangial expansion did not affect the final GFR.

Therefore, from above information, there are several histological parameters, which were associated with renal functional changes. Further longitudinal studies, which handle larger cohorts of types 1 and 2 diabetes, are necessary to elucidate histological changes as cause or result for the renal functional changes.

8.4 The Importance of Serial Renal Biopsy

In fact, we need to perform research-related serial renal biopsy to elucidate what histological factors affect on renal functional changes (cause or results?). However, it is difficult to perform research-related serial renal biopsy, both in types 1 and 2 diabetes. Previously, in 11 normo- and microalbuminuric patients with type 1 diabetes, the urinary albumin excretion was found to increase in parallel with mesangial expansion over an interval of 5.6 ± 1.6 years [13] using serial renal biopsy. However,

Table 8.3 Clinical characteristics, renal function, and morphometric data in patients with IAH ≥ 2.0 and IAH < 2.0

	IAH ≥ 2.0	IAH < 2.0	*P*-value
Sex (M/F)	7 (5/2)	22 (17/5)	ND
Age (years)	48 ± 12	49 ± 10	0.765
Known duration of diabetes (years)	12 ± 8	12 ± 7	0.955
HbA_{1c} (%) [mmol/mol]	8.2 ± 1.7 [66.0 ± 8.1]	8.3 ± 2.0 [66.9 ± 4.6]	0.924
UAE at baseline (μg/min)	48.6 (7.3–82.4)	12.2 (0.0–180.2)	0.161
UAE at follow-up (μg/min)	93.1 (3.4–1180.3)	14.0 (1.3–442.2)	0.208
P-value (UAE at baseline vs. follow-up)	0.157	0.231	–
Iohexol-GFR at baseline (ml/min/1.73 m^2)	122.6 ± 28.1	117.3 ± 27.1	0.657
Iohexol-GFR at follow-up (ml/min/1.73 m^2)	77.2 ± 36.2	112.9 ± 21.8	0.005
P-value (GFR at baseline vs. follow-up)	0.025	0.443	–
MGV ($\times 10^6$ μm^3)	2.6 ± 0.4	3.3 ± 0.8	0.091
Vv(Int/cortex)	0.20 ± 0.05	0.21 ± 0.04	0.600
%GS	8.1 ± 13.4	3.9 ± 9.6	0.488
GBM width (nm)	721 ± 127	708 ± 112	0.823
Vv(Mes/glom)	0.27 ± 0.07	0.24 ± 0.07	0.302
Sv(PGBM/glom) ($\mu m^2/\mu m^3$)	0.10 ± 0.02	0.11 ± 0.04	0.370
Total Mes/glom ($\times 10^6$ μm^3)	0.71 ± 0.34	0.77 ± 0.26	0.638
Filtration S/G (μm^2)	0.26 ± 0.04	0.37 ± 0.15	0.124

Data are *n*, median (interquartile range), or means ± SD

UAE urinary albumin excretion rate, *GFR* glomerular filtration rate, *MGV* mean glomerular volume, *Vv(Int/cortex)* volume fraction of cortical interstitium, *%GS* percent of global glomerular sclerosis, *GBM* glomerular basement membrane width, *Vv(Mes/glom)* volume fraction of mesangium, *Sv(PGBM/glom)* surface density of peripheral GBM per glomerulus, *Total Mes/glom* total mesangium per glomerulus; *Filtration S/G* filtration surface per glomerulus, *ND* not done for selection criterion

Table 8.4 Stepwise regression analysis (dependent variable: final GFR)

Independent variables	*F*	*P*
MGV	2.31	0.147
Vv(Int/cortex)	1.60	0.223
%GS	1.68	0.211
IAH	5.20	0.036
GBM width	0.24	0.629
Vv(Mes/glom)	2.78	0.113
Sv(PGBM/glom)	1.58	0.226

GFR glomerular filtration rate, *MGV* mean glomerular volume, *Vv(Int/cortex)* interstitial volume fraction, *%GS* percent global glomerular sclerosis, *IAH* index of arteriolar hyalinosis, *GBM* glomerular basement membrane, *Vv(Mes/glom)* mesangial volume fraction, *Sv(PGBM/glom)* surface density of peripheral GBM

that study did not describe relationships between the renal histological parameters and the decline in the renal function over the long term. Another report on 18 microalbuminuric patients with type 1 diabetes showed that urinary albumin excretion was correlated with the mesangial matrix/glomerular volume fraction in the follow-up biopsy, but no changes in the renal function were described during 2–3 years of follow-up [27]. A longer observational study showed that only the mean of HbA1c value affected the GFR at the end of the 8-year study, while no histological parameters had any effect [28]. Another study noted that a change in renal interstitial fibrosis was a risk factor for a loss of renal function during 4 years of follow-up [29]; however, that study only examined diabetic patients with macroalbuminuria (type 1 diabetes, $n = 29$; type 2 diabetes, $n = 19$) and did not include any patients with normoalbuminuria or microalbuminuria. A very old Japanese study [30] revealed relationships between glycemic control and changes in the renal histology using serial renal biopsy. However, the study [30] did not describe the type of diabetes or provide details about the renal function at the follow-up examination. Thus, to the best of our knowledge, although research regarding the course of the renal structural-functional relationships was planned in order to elucidate the natural history of diabetic nephropathy in type 1 diabetes [31], there is little information regarding the relationships between the changes in the renal histology and the functional changes that occur in diabetes patients over the long-term period. The effects of renin-angiotensin-aldosterone blockade on retinal and renal changes have been shown by serial biopsy [32]; however, that report did not show the detailed relationships between the changes in the renal histology and function over a long observational period. Recently, research-related serial renal biopsies were performed in normo- and microalbuminuric Japanese type 2 diabetic patients [33]. The study revealed that the decreases in the GFR in patients with type 2 diabetes with normo- or microalbuminuria at baseline were associated with a decreased glomerular filtration surface, as a result of mesangial expansion during a mean 6 years of observation (Fig. 8.7a, b). However, the phenomenon should be examined in larger number of patients with longer duration. Thus, the histological findings that cause a decline in the renal function or an increase in albuminuria in patients with types 1 and 2 diabetes remain unknown.

8.5 The Relationships Between Diabetic Nephropathy Lesions and Retinopathy

A classical diagnosis of diabetic nephropathy without renal biopsy is made as the following criteria: (1) A patient has diabetes with at least 5-year duration. (2) Microalbuminuria or macroalbuminuria is present. (3) No massive hematuria or bacteriuria is present. (4) A patient has diabetic retinopathy. (5) A patient has no history of other renal disease than diabetic nephropathy. Therefore, information regarding diabetic retinopathy is clinically very important to diagnose diabetic

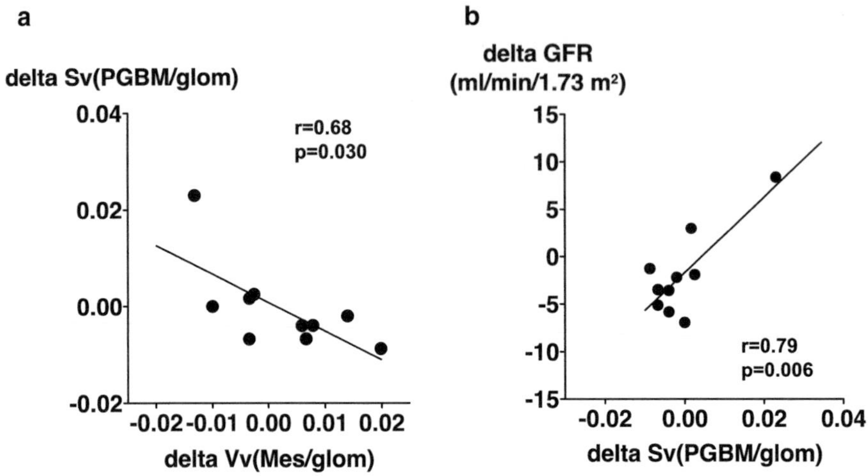

Fig. 8.7 The relationship of change in Sv(PGBM/glom) with change in Vv(Mes/glom) (**a**) and change in GFR (**b**). The annual change in the Sv(PGBM/glom) was negatively correlated with that of the Vv(Mes/glom) ($r = 0.68$, $P = 0.030$) during 6 years of follow-up (**a**). In addition, the annual decrease in the Sv(PGBM/glom) was positively correlated with the decrease in the GFR over the 6 years after the initial renal biopsy ($r = 0.79$, $P = 0.006$) (**b**)

nephropathy since there may be a relationship between diabetic retinopathy and nephropathy. In fact, the patients with diabetic retinopathy had significant increases in the mesangial volume fraction as revealed by electron microscopic morphometry compared with that in patients without diabetic retinopathy [34]. In addition, clear relationship between diabetic retinopathy and urinary albumin excretion has been described in Caucasian type 2 diabetic patients [35, 36]. These data suggested that typical diabetic glomerulosclerosis and renal histological severity related to diabetic retinopathy in patients with type 2 diabetes and were compatible with that seen in patients with type 1 diabetes with diabetic retinopathy.

On the other hand, Chavers et al. [37] also indicated that severity of diabetic retinopathy is concordant with increased Vv(Mes/glom) and decreased Sv(PGBM/glom) in Caucasian type 1 diabetic patients. However, they also showed that 27% of these patients had advanced diabetic retinopathy with normal Vv(Mes/glom). Recently, it has been shown that severity of diabetic nephropathy lesions might be in part discordant to diabetic retinopathy grade [38, 39]. Kanauchi et al. [38] performed renal biopsy in 221 Japanese type 2 diabetic patients to examine the relationship between diabetic nephropathy and retinopathy. In that study, five patients had advanced diabetic glomerulosclerosis without diabetic retinopathy although concordance between diabetic nephropathy and retinopathy was shown in these Japanese patients as a group. The study showed that there were some patients with diabetic nephropathy without diabetic retinopathy although proteinuria in diabetic patients without diabetic retinopathy was usually thought to be nondiabetic origins.

In another report [39], renal biopsy was performed in 36 type 2 diabetic patients with clinical proteinuria to examine the relationships between diabetic nephropathy and retinopathy. The report described that diabetic patients with nodular glomerulosclerosis had more severe diabetic retinopathy than those with mesangial sclerosis alone. However, almost half of the patients with mesangial sclerosis alone had no diabetic retinopathy in the study. Thus, the authors suggested that nodular lesions and mesangial expansion be caused by different pathogenesis. These results suggest that there is discordance between diabetic nephropathy and retinopathy in type 2 diabetes. However, one of these reports [39] used only overt nephropathic patients, and there is no description of albuminuria in another [38]. Previous reports [11], which showed structural heterogeneity in Caucasian microalbuminuric type 2 diabetes, indicated that proliferative diabetic retinopathy was seen only in the patients with typical diabetic glomerulosclerosis.

Previously, it was shown that the type 2 diabetic patients with concomitant microalbuminuria and diabetic retinopathy had progressive renal function decline [40]. However, it is still unknown whether or not the CII pattern, the presence of diabetic retinopathy, and microalbuminuria are related to each other and which combinations affect renal function decline. Therefore, we analyzed the course of renal function in normoalbuminuric and microalbuminuric patients with the CII pattern and diabetic retinopathy (Table 8.5) [41]. Noteworthy, all of the normoalbuminuric patients and seven of eight microalbuminuric patients with the CII pattern had diabetic retinopathy among all the patients (Table 8.5). There were no significant differences in any of the morphometric data between the two groups, and baseline GFR did not differ between the two groups. After 7.1 ± 3.8 years of follow-up,

Table 8.5 Follow-up data of renal function between normoalbuminuria and microalbuminuria with typical histological injury patterns and diabetic retinopathy

	Normoalbuminuria with CII	Microalbuminuria with CII	*P*-value
Number	5	7	ND
DR	5	7	ND
UAE at baseline (μg/min)	5.4 (5.1–14.6)	48.6 (28.3–52.0)	ND
UAE at follow-up (μg/min)	15.4 (4.6–244.0)	71.9 (24.4–428.3)	ND
P-value (UAE at baseline vs. follow-up)	0.834	0.848	
Iohexol-GFR at baseline (ml/min/1.73 m^2)	107.3 ± 19.8	130.6 ± 54.7	0.925
Iohexol-GFR at follow-up (ml/min/1.73 m^2)	120.6 ± 23.4	80.9 ± 42.0	0.309
P-value (GFR at baseline vs. follow-up)	0.821	0.048	

Data are *n*, median (interquartile range), or means ± SD

UAE urinary albumin excretion, *GFR* glomerular filtration rate, *ND* not done for selection criterion

Table 8.6 Stepwise regression analysis

Independent variables (Final GFR)	*F*-value	*P*-value
Vv(Mes/glom)	3.360	0.08
DR only	0.708	0.41
Microalbuminuria only	2.766	0.11
Histological injury pattern only	1.934	0.18
DR and microalbuminuria	7.240	0.01

GFR glomerular filtration rate, *Vv(Mes/glom)* volume fraction of mesangium, *DR* diabetic retinopathy

urinary albumin excretion did not change from baseline to follow-up in either group. However, GFR in microalbuminuria with CII had significantly decreased compared to the baseline, while GFR did not change from baseline to follow-up in normoalbuminuria with the CII pattern (Table 8.5).

The stepwise regression analysis showed that the categorization using both diabetic retinopathy and microalbuminuria mostly affected GFR at the final observation (Table 8.6). The categorization of the presence of only diabetic retinopathy, or only microalbuminuria, or mesangial expansion, did not significantly affect the final GFR (Table 8.6).

We need to perform careful longitudinal study to elucidate the course and relationships between diabetic nephropathy and retinopathy both in types 1 and 2 diabetes.

8.6 Similarity or Difference of Diabetic Nephropathy Between Types 1 and 2 Diabetes

Table 8.7 shows the similarity or difference of diabetic nephropathy lesions and association with clinical parameters between types 1 and 2 diabetic patients especially at early stage (normo-microalbuminuria) of diabetic nephropathy. Basic histological findings of glomerulus, tubulointerstitium, and arterioles are almost same between 2 types of diabetes. The most important difference is that there is histological heterogeneity of renal tissues at early stage of diabetic nephropathy [11, 24]. This phenomenon might be one of the causes of the lack of renal structural-functional relationships especially with albuminuria in type 2 diabetic patients. The detailed relationships of diabetic nephropathy lesions with other diabetic complications, i.e., diabetic retinopathy, are still unknown.

In conclusion, we need to elucidate histological parameters, which predict renal function loss, and further longitudinal study using serial biopsy is needed to elucidate detailed renal structural-functional relationships at early stage of diabetic nephropathy in both types of diabetes.

Table 8.7 Similarity or difference of diabetic nephropathy between types 1 and 2 diabetes

Characteristic of histology		Type 1 diabetes	Type 2 diabetes
Basic histological findings		GBM thickening, mesangial expansion, tubulointerstitial expansion, TBM thickening, arteriolar hyalinosis	Same as left
Histological heterogeneity		Almost absent	Striking
Renal structural-functional relationships	vs. albuminuria	Present	Absent at early stage of albuminuria
	vs. GFR	Glomerular filtration surface shows positive correlation	Almost same as left
Predictors for renal functional decline		GBM thickening, mesangial expansion	GBM thickening, Mesangial expansion, Arteriolar hyalinosis
Association with diabetic retinopathy lesions		Mesangial expansion degree associated with diabetic retinopathy severity	Might be present under typical diabetic glomerulosclerosis
Serial biopsy findings with renal function		Present for albuminuria	Might be present, should be clarified in large number of cases

References

1. Caramori ML, Fioretto P, Mauer M. Low glomerular filtration rate in normoalbuminuric type 1 diabetic patients: an indicator of more advanced glomerular lesions. Diabetes. 2003;52(4):1036–40.
2. Ekinci EI, Jerums G, Skene A, et al. Renal structure in normoalbuminuric and albuminuric patients with type 2 diabetes and impaired renal function. Diabetes Care. 2013;36(11):3620–6.
3. Mauer SM, Steffes MW, Ellis EN, Sutherland DE, Brown DM, Goetz FC. Structural-functional relationships in diabetic nephropathy. J Clin Invest. 1984;74(4):1143–55.
4. Lane PH, Steffes MW, Fioretto P, Mauer SM. Renal interstitial expansion in insulin-dependent diabetes mellitus. Kidney Int. 1993;43(3):661–7.
5. Jensen EB, Gundersen HJ, Osterby R. Determination of membrane thickness distribution from orthogonal intercepts. J Microsc. 1979;115(1):19–33.
6. Fioretto P, Steffes MW, Mauer M. Glomerular structure in nonproteinuric IDDM patients with various levels of albuminuria. Diabetes. 1994;43(11):1358–64.
7. Weibel ER. Morphometry of the human lung: the state of the art after two decades. Bull Eur Physiopathol Respir. 1979;15(5):999–1013.
8. Harris RD, Steffes MW, Bilous RW, Sutherland DE, Mauer SM. Global glomerular sclerosis and glomerular arteriolar hyalinosis in insulin dependent diabetes. Kidney Int. 1991;40(1):107–14.
9. Drummond K, Mauer M, International Diabetic Nephropathy Study Group. The early natural history of nephropathy in type 1 diabetes: II. Early renal structural changes in type 1 diabetes. Diabetes. 2002;51(5):1580–7.
10. Moriya T, Omura K, Matsubara M, Yoshida Y, Hayama K, Ouchi M. Arteriolar hyalinosis predicts increase in albuminuria and GFR decline in normo- and microalbuminuric japanese patients with type 2 diabetes. Diabetes Care. 2017;40(10):1373–8.
11. Fioretto P, Mauer M, Brocco E, et al. Patterns of renal injury in NIDDM patients with microalbuminuria. Diabetologia. 1996;39(12):1569–76.

12. Moriya T, Moriya R, Yajima Y, Steffes MW, Mauer M. Urinary albumin as an indicator of diabetic nephropathy lesions in Japanese type 2 diabetic patients. Nephron. 2002;91(2):292–9.
13. Fioretto P, Steffes MW, Sutherland DE, Mauer M. Sequential renal biopsies in insulin-dependent diabetic patients: structural factors associated with clinical progression. Kidney Int. 1995;48(6):1929–35.
14. Caramori ML, Parks A, Mauer M. Renal lesions predict progression of diabetic nephropathy in type 1 diabetes. J Am Soc Nephrol. 2013;24(7):1175–81.
15. Ellis EN, Steffes MW, Goetz FC, Sutherland DE, Mauer SM. Glomerular filtration surface in type I diabetes mellitus. Kidney Int. 1986;29(4):889–94.
16. Moriya T, Tsuchiya A, Okizaki S, Hayashi A, Tanaka K, Shichiri M. Glomerular hyperfiltration and increased glomerular filtration surface are associated with renal function decline in normo- and microalbuminuric type 2 diabetes. Kidney Int. 2012;81(5):486–93.
17. Caramori ML, Kim Y, Huang C, et al. Cellular basis of diabetic nephropathy: 1. Study design and renal structural-functional relationships in patients with long-standing type 1 diabetes. Diabetes. 2002;51(2):506–13.
18. Moriya T, Tanaka K, Hosaka T, Hirasawa Y, Fujita Y. Renal structure as an indicator for development of albuminuria in normo- and microalbuminuric type 2 diabetic patients. Diabetes Res Clin Pract. 2008;82(3):298–304.
19. Nosadini R, Velussi M, Brocco E, et al. Course of renal function in type 2 diabetic patients with abnormalities of albumin excretion rate. Diabetes. 2000;49(3):476–84.
20. Fufaa GD, Weil EJ, Lemley KV, et al. Structural predictors of loss of renal function in American Indians with type 2 diabetes. Clin J Am Soc Nephrol. 2016;11(2):254–61.
21. Mise K, Hoshino J, Ueno T, et al. Prognostic value of tubulointerstitial lesions, urinary N-acetyl-beta-d-glucosaminidase, and urinary beta2-microglobulin in patients with type 2 diabetes and biopsy-proven diabetic nephropathy. Clin J Am Soc Nephrol. 2016;11(4):593–601.
22. Shimizu M, Furuichi K, Toyama T, et al. Long-term outcomes of Japanese type 2 diabetic patients with biopsy-proven diabetic nephropathy. Diabetes Care. 2013;36(11):3655–62.
23. Li L, Zhang X, Li Z, et al. Renal pathological implications in type 2 diabetes mellitus patients with renal involvement. J Diabetes Complicat. 2016;31(1):114–21.
24. Moriya T, Suzuki Y, Inomata S, Iwano M, Kanauchi M, Haneda M. Renal histological heterogeneity and functional progress in normoalbuminuric and microalbuminuric Japanese patients with type 2 diabetes. BMJ Open Diabetes Res Care. 2014;2(1):e000029.
25. Myers BD, Nelson RG, Williams GW, et al. Glomerular function in Pima Indians with noninsulin-dependent diabetes mellitus of recent onset. J Clin Invest. 1991;88(2):524–30.
26. Li L, Zhang X, Li Z, et al. Renal pathological implications in type 2 diabetes mellitus patients with renal involvement. J Diabetes Complicat. 2017;31(1):114–21.
27. Bangstad HJ, Osterby R, Dahl-Jorgensen K, Berg KJ, Hartmann A, Hanssen KF. Improvement of blood glucose control in IDDM patients retards the progression of morphological changes in early diabetic nephropathy. Diabetologia. 1994;37(5):483–90.
28. Bangstad HJ, Osterby R, Rudberg S, Hartmann A, Brabrand K, Hanssen KF. Kidney function and glomerulopathy over 8 years in young patients with Type I (insulin-dependent) diabetes mellitus and microalbuminuria. Diabetologia. 2002;45(2):253–61.
29. Taft JL, Nolan CJ, Yeung SP, Hewitson TD, Martin FI. Clinical and histological correlations of decline in renal function in diabetic patients with proteinuria. Diabetes. 1994;43(8):1046–51.
30. Takazakura E, Nakamoto Y, Hayakawa H, Kawai K, Muramoto S. Onset and progression of diabetic glomerulosclerosis; a prospective study based on serial renal biopsies. Diabetes. 1975;24(1):1–9.
31. Mauer M, Drummond K. The early natural history of nephropathy in type 1 diabetes: I. Study design and baseline characteristics of the study participants. Diabetes. 2002;51(5):1572–9.
32. Mauer M, Zinman B, Gardiner R, et al. Renal and retinal effects of enalapril and losartan in type 1 diabetes. N Engl J Med. 2009;361(1):40–51.
33. Moriya T, Yamagishi T, Matsubara M, Ouchi M. Serial renal biopsies in normo- and microalbuminuric patients with type 2 diabetes demonstrate that loss of renal function is associated

with a reduction in glomerular filtration surface secondary to mesangial expansion. J Diabetes Complicat. 2019;33(5):368–73.
34. Klein R, Zinman B, Gardiner R, et al. The relationship of diabetic retinopathy to preclinical diabetic glomerulopathy lesions in type 1 diabetic patients: the Renin-Angiotensin System Study. Diabetes. 2005;54(2):527–33.
35. Schmitz A, Vaeth M. Microalbuminuria: a major risk factor in non-insulin-dependent diabetes. A 10-year follow-up study of 503 patients. Diabet Med. 1988;5(2):126–34.
36. Marshall SM, Alberti KG. Comparison of the prevalence and associated features of abnormal albumin excretion in insulin-dependent and non-insulin-dependent diabetes. Q J Med. 1989;70(261):61–71.
37. Chavers BM, Mauer SM, Ramsay RC, Steffes MW. Relationship between retinal and glomerular lesions in IDDM patients. Diabetes. 1994;43(3):441–6.
38. Kanauchi M, Kawano T, Uyama H, Shiiki H, Dohi K. Discordance between retinopathy and nephropathy in type 2 diabetes. Nephron. 1998;80(2):171–4.
39. Schwartz MM, Lewis EJ, Leonard-Martin T, Lewis JB, Batlle D. Renal pathology patterns in type II diabetes mellitus: relationship with retinopathy. The Collaborative Study Group. Nephrol Dial Transplant. 1998;13(10):2547–52.
40. Moriya T, Tanaka S, Kawasaki R, et al. Diabetic retinopathy and microalbuminuria can predict macroalbuminuria and renal function decline in Japanese type 2 diabetic patients: Japan Diabetes Complications Study. Diabetes Care. 2013;36(9):2803–9.
41. Moriya T, Matsubara M, Kishihara E, Yoshida Y, Ouchi M. Type 2 diabetic patients with diabetic retinopathy and concomitant microalbuminuria showed typical diabetic glomerulosclerosis and progressive renal dysfunction. J Diabetes Complicat. 2016;30(6):1111–6.

Chapter 9
Study at AMED Collecting 600 Biopsy-Proven Diabetic Nephropathies

Kengo Furuichi

9.1 Clinical and Pathological Backgrounds of Diabetic Nephropathy

Diabetic nephropathy (DN) is one of the three major complications of diabetes; it is a microangiopathy caused by hyperglycemia. In a typical case, it begins with microalbuminuria and then progresses to end-stage kidney failure after exacerbation of proteinuria and reduction in kidney function. Until now, DN, particularly early nephropathy, is diagnosed with the detection of microalbuminuria. Therefore, detection of small amount of albuminuria is important for an early diagnosis. Urine albumin should be measured in protein-negative or slightly protein-positive cases.

In general, it would be acceptable that the major characteristic pathological changes in the kidneys in diabetic patients are observed in the glomeruli. Moreover, diffuse lesions can be observed as initial changes, and the characteristic nodular lesion, Kimmelstiel–Wilson lesion, is detected in advanced cases. Finally, the pathological changes end with glomerulosclerosis. However, the onset and progression pattern of kidney dysfunction and proteinuria greatly vary with each case [1–3]. Classification of the risks involved in the development and progression of kidney disease is therefore crucial. Additionally, improvement in blood glucose control, use of renin–angiotensin blockers, and an increase in the aging population have changed the clinical manifestation of kidney disease in diabetic patients. Therefore, the pathological changes of each diabetic case should greatly vary, and it would be important to evaluate the pathological changes of each case.

For a therapeutic approach toward diabetes with kidney disease cases, risk classification with clinical and pathological findings would be beneficial. The Japanese classification of DN is a clinical classification based on albuminuria and estimated

K. Furuichi (✉)
Department of Nephrology, Kanazawa Medical University, Uchinada, Japan
e-mail: furuichi@kanazawa-med.ac.jp

T. Wada et al. (eds.), *Diabetic Kidney Disease*,
https://doi.org/10.1007/978-981-15-9301-7_9

glomerular filtration rate (eGFR) [4, 5]. Along with this clinical classification, pathological findings are also important prognostic factors for kidney diseases [6]. Moreover, kidney biopsy must be performed to exclude other kidney diseases besides diabetes. Recent meta-analysis on studies of kidney biopsies in diabetic cases revealed an extremely variable change of kidney diseases [7]. Furthermore, recent autopsy studies revealed that pathological changes of DN developed before the onset of clinical findings such as albuminuria and decreasing eGFR [8–11]. Accordingly, evaluation of pathological changes of kidney disease in diabetic cases becomes clinically important. However, in general clinical practice, a kidney biopsy is rarely performed in diabetic cases demonstrating a typical diabetic clinical course of proteinuria and kidney dysfunction.

9.2 Importance of Pathological Findings in Diabetic Nephropathy

As described in previous section, the pathological manifestations of DN in type 2 diabetes are diverse [12, 13]. Therefore, precise evaluation of pathological evaluation for each case is required. A previous study indicated that some pathological findings were good predictors of kidney events, cardiovascular events, and all-cause mortality [6, 14]. Nodular lesions and mesangiolysis were characteristic pathological findings of DN and have been reported as predictive markers of improper renal function [6, 15, 16]. An exudative lesion is also a typical pathological change in DN. A previous study indicated that patients without exudative lesions had a significantly better renal survival rate than those with such lesions [17]. However, it is also reported that advanced diabetic kidney lesions were incidentally detected even in normoalbuminuric cases [15]. These pathological observations of heterogeneity in diabetic kidney disease indicated that evaluating pathological findings and clinical categorization could assist in predicting kidney prognosis, cardiovascular events, and all-cause mortality in DN patients.

9.3 A Pathological Classification by the Renal Pathology Society of the United States for Diabetic Nephropathy

A set of definitions and classifications of pathological findings for DN was published by the Renal Pathology Society of the United States [18], and the classification of a glomerular lesion is mainly based on the mesangial expansion of DN (Table 9.1). Other pathological findings such as thickening of the glomerular basement membrane, nodular lesion, and glomerulosclerosis are additional grading factors. This classification of a glomerular lesion is classified into five grades: I, IIA, IIB, III, and IV. There is no evacuation for each glomerular pathological lesion, such

Table 9.1 The pathological classification system of Renal Pathological Society

<table>
<tr><td>Glomerular lesions</td><td colspan="2">GScl > 50% (class IV)
↓
Nodular (class III)
↓
Mesangial expansion > 50%
(Diffuse)(class IIB,IIA)
↓
Glomerular basement membrane thickening by electron microscopy (class I)</td></tr>
<tr><td>Interstitial lesions</td><td>Interstitial fibrosis and tubular atrophy</td><td>0 (no IFTA)
1 (<25%)
2 (25–50%)
3 (≧50%)</td></tr>
<tr><td></td><td>Interstitial cell infiltration</td><td>0 (no infiltration), 1 (infiltration only in relation to IFTA), 2 (infiltration in areas without IFTA)</td></tr>
<tr><td>Vascular lesions</td><td>Arteriolar hyalinosis</td><td>0 (no hyalinosis)
1 (at least one area of arteriolar hyalinosis)
2 (more than one area of arteriolar hyalinosis)</td></tr>
<tr><td></td><td>Arteriosclerosis</td><td>Intimal thickening greater than thickness of media
0 (no intimal thickening)
1 (intimal thickening less than thickness of media)
2 (intimal thickening greater than thickness of media)</td></tr>
</table>

GScl global glomerulosclerosis, *IFTA* interstitial fibrosis and tubular atrophy

as nodular lesion, exudative lesion, mesangiolysis etc. Conversely, interstitial and vascular pathological lesions are evaluated individually. Interstitial fibrosis and renal tubular atrophy (IFTA), interstitial cell infiltration, arteriolar hyalinosis, and arteriosclerosis are individually assessed (Table 9.1). The pathological classification of DN by the Renal Pathology Society of the United States is systematic and organized, predicting renal outcomes in DN patients [17–19]. However, this classification omitted some important pathological findings, particularly regarding glomerular lesions.

9.4 A New Pathological Classification for Diabetic Nephropathy

A new pathological classification for DN is published under support from the Ministry of Health, Labor and Welfare of Japan and AMED [20–22] (Table 9.2). In contrast to the classification by the Renal Pathology Society of the United States, this new classification has nine glomerular lesions: diffuse lesion (mesangial

Table 9.2 A new pathological classification for DN in AMED study

Glomerular lesions	Diffuse	0 normal or mild mesangial expansion 1 mesangial expansion ≦ capillary lumen 2 mesangial expansion = capillary lumen 3 mesangial expansion ≧ capillary lumen
	Nodular	0 (no nodular lesion), 1 (one or more nodular lesions in all biopsy specimens, not care of nodular size)
	SubendW	Double contour of basement membrane (%) 0 (<10%), 1 (10–25%), 2 (25–50%), 3 (≧50%)
	Exudative	0 (not detected) 1 (detected one or more lesions in all biopsy specimens)
	MesLy	0 (not detected) 1 (detected one or more lesions in all biopsy specimens)
	PVas	0 (not detected) 1 (detected one or more lesions in all biopsy specimens)
	GScl	(number of global glomerulosclerosis and collapsing glomerulopathy ・ ischemic nephropathy)/number of all glomeruli (%)
	SScl	Number of segmental glomerulosclerosis/number of all glomerulus (%)
	GMeg	More than 250 μm in glomerular diameter 0 (not detected), 1 (detected)
Interstitial lesions	IFTA	0 (no IFTA), 1 (<25%), 2 (25–50%), 3 (≧50%)
	ICell	0 (no cell infiltration), 1 (<25%), 2 (25–50%), 3 (≧50%)
Vascular lesions	Hyalin	0 (no hyalinosis) 1 (one or more partial arterioral hyalinosis) 2 (around 50% hyalinosis) 3 (more than 50% hyalinosis or penetrating hyalinosis)
	Arterio	0 (no intimal thickening) 1 (intimal thickness/media thickness < 1) 2 (intimal thickening and intimal thickness/media thickness ≧ 1) EVG staining is helpful for determination

Diffuse: diffuse lesion (mesangial expansion), Nodular: nodular lesion (nodular sclerosis), SubendW: subendothelial space widening (double contour of basement membrane), Exudative: exudative lesion, MesLy: mesangiolysis/microaneurysm, PVas: peri-hilar neovascularization (polar vasculosis), GScl: global glomerulosclerosis/collapsing glomerular change · ischemic glomerular change, SScl: segmental glomerulosclerosis, GMeg: glomerulomegaly, IFTA: interstitial fibrosis and tubular atrophy, ICell: interstitial cell infiltration, Hyalin: arteriolar hyalinosis, Arterio: arteriosclerosis with intimal thickening

expansion), nodular lesion (nodular sclerosis), subendothelial space widening (double contour of basement membrane), exudative lesion, mesangiolysis/microaneurysm, peri-hilar neovascularization (polar vasculosis), global glomerulosclerosis/collapsing glomerular change, ischemic glomerular change, and segmental glomerulosclerosis. Regarding interstitial lesions, this new classification is similar to the classification of the Renal Pathology Society of the United States. These are four interstitial and vascular lesions: IFTA, interstitial cell infiltration, arteriolar hyalinosis, and arteriosclerosis with intimal thickening.

9.5 Definition of Each Pathological Finding and Score

The detailed points on each definition and score were published as a handbook [20]. Following is a simple summary of the definition of each finding, and the scores are shown in Table 9.2.

Diffuse Lesion (Mesangial Expansion)
A diffuse lesion is defined as mesangial matrix expansion that is double the width of the nucleus of a mesangial cell. The lesion should be detected in at least two peripheral lobules in one glomerulus.

Nodular Lesion (Nodular Sclerosis)
A nodular lesion is defined as a rounded mesangial matrix expansion where no normal capillary is present.

Supportive findings: A typical nodular lesion exhibits low PAM and periodic acid–Schiff (PAS) staining. Uptake with PAM and PAS should be standardized by arterial media. A low PAM and PAS staining area is usually blue with Masson's trichrome staining. The difference between diffuse and nodular lesions is the presence of normal capillaries around a diffuse lesion and the absence of normal capillaries around a nodular lesion.

Subendothelial Space Widening
Edematous widening of the subendothelial space indicated subendothelial space widening.

Exudative Lesion
An exudative lesion is defined by serum amorphous protein deposits in the subendothelial space (fibrin cap) or Bowman's capsule wall (capsular drop).

Mesangiolysis/Microaneurysm
Mesangiolysis is defined as dissolution or attenuation of the mesangial matrix and degeneration of mesangial cells.

Peri-Hilar Neovascularization
There is neovascularization in the glomerular hilar region around the afferent and efferent arterioles, and the vascular wall often has hyalinosis.

Global Glomerulosclerosis, Collapsing Glomerulopathy, and Ischemic Nephropathy
All the glomerulocapillaries are sclerosed, the capillary lumen is not detected, and the glomerulocapillaries are collapsing.

Segmental Glomerulosclerosis
In segmental glomerulosclerosis, part of the glomerulocapillaries is sclerosed.

Glomerulomegaly
In glomerulomegaly, one or more glomerular diameter is greater than 250 μm in all biopsy specimens. In 400× visual field microscopy, the glomerular diameter is usually around 500 μm.

Interstitial Fibrosis, IFTA
Interstitial fibrosis is defined as the accumulation of collagen and related molecules in the interstitium. Tubular atrophy is defined as a decrease in tubular diameter and number.

Interstitial Cell Infiltration
Interstitial cell infiltration is defined as the accumulation of inflammatory cell infiltration the interstitium.

Arteriolar Hyalinosis
This is the ratio of hyaline thickness to whole arteriolar wall thickness expressed as a percentage. A totally occluded artery and an artery connecting to a globally sclerotic glomerulus are shown for comparison.

Intimal Thickening
Fibrous intimal thickening of an arteriole or larger artery (interlobular artery arcuate artery) should be evaluated together with the symmetrical wall. Advanced intimal thickening is dominant in some patients and the media is hard to detect. The branching artery is not evaluated.

9.6 Pathological Findings Based on the Classification of Diabetic Nephropathy in Japan

9.6.1 The Classification of Diabetic Nephropathy in Japan

The Japanese classification of DN was published in 2014 by the Joint Committee on Diabetes Nephropathy (Japanese Society of Nephrology, Japan Diabetes Society, Japanese Society for Dialysis Therapy, and Japan Society of Metabolism and Clinical Nutrition) [4, 5] (Table 9.3). DN was classified according to the levels of albuminuria and eGFR, because these determine kidney prognosis, cardiovascular events, and all-cause mortality in Japanese diabetic kidney disease patients.

9.6.2 Kidney Biopsy Cohort in Japan

With support from the Ministry of Health, Labour and Welfare in Japan and the Japan Agency for Medical Research and Development (AMED), 600 kidney biopsies from diabetic cases were collected from 13 facilities throughout Japan and analyzed [22]. A median observation period is 70.4 months. The mean age was 57.8 years old, and 67% of the patients were male. The mean systolic and diastolic BP

Table 9.3 Classification of diabetic nephropathy 2014 in Japan

Stage	Urinary albumin (mg/g Cr) or urinary protein (g/g Cr)	GFR (eGFR) (mL/min/1.73 m²)
Stage 1 (pre-nephropathy)	Normoalbuminuria (<30)	≥30[a]
Stage 2 (incipient nephropathy)	Microalbuminuria (30–299)[b]	≥30
Stage 3 (overt nephropathy)	Macroalbuminuria (≥300) or Persistent proteinuria (≥0.5)	≥30[c]
Stage 4 (kidney failure)	Any albuminuria/proteinuria status[d]	<30
Stage 5 (dialysis therapy)	Any status on continued dialysis therapy	

[a]While a GFR of less than 60 mL/min/1.73 m² is consistent with the diagnosis of CKD, underlying causes other than diabetic nephropathy may be involved in patients with a GFR below 60 mL/min/1.73 m², thus calling for the differential diagnosis between diabetic nephropathy and any other potential nondiabetic kidney diseases

[b]Patients with microalbuminuria are to be diagnosed as incipient nephropathy after the differential diagnosis based on the criteria for an early diagnosis of diabetic nephropathy

[c]Precautions are required in patients with macroalbuminuria, in whom renal events (e.g., a decrease in eGFR to half its baseline value, the need for dialysis) have been shown to increase as the GFR decreases below 60 mL/min/1.73 m²

[d]All patients with a GFR of less than 30 mL/min/1.73 m² are classified as exhibiting kidney failure, regardless of their urinary albumin/protein values. However, in those with normoalbuminuria and microalbuminuria, the differential diagnosis is required between diabetic nephropathy and any other potential nondiabetic kidney diseases

were 144.5 and 78.9 mmHg, respectively. The mean serum Alb was 3.3 mg/dL, and HbA1c was 7.6%. This is one of the biggest biopsy cohort with long observation clinical data of diabetic nephropathy in the world.

9.7 Characteristic Pathological Findings Based on the Classification of Diabetic Nephropathy in Japan

In the overall analysis, the pathological scores for glomerular, interstitial, and vascular lesions were higher in the higher stages and were the highest in stage 4 (Table 9.4, Fig. 9.1). The scores of each pathological finding correlated strongly with that of other pathological findings. These findings indicate that pathological changes of diabetic nephropathy progress in accordance with the progression of clinical manifestation in analysis of mass study. Moreover, each pathological change progresses in a parallel with other pathological changes in accordance with the progression of clinical stages. Although these findings are speculative, this study clearly showed the data.

In addition to this overall analysis, subanalysis based on similar clinical manifestation is valuable and important. In an analysis based on DN classification in Japan, each stage had specific characteristic pathological findings. Even in stage 1, 78% of the

Table 9.4 Mean score of each pathological findings

	Stage 1	Stage 2	Stage 3	Stage 4	Total
Diffuse	1.2	1.5	2.2	2.5	2.1
Nodular	0.1	0.2	0.5	0.6	0.4
SubendW	0.4	0.7	1.1	1.4	1.0
Exudative	0.1	0.2	0.5	0.6	0.5
MesLy	0.1	0.2	0.5	0.5	0.4
PVas	0.2	0.7	0.8	0.8	0.7
GScl (%)	7.9	13.0	25.0	40.0	24.4
SScl (%)	3.0	1.6	3.8	5.7	3.8
GMeg	0.1	0.3	0.4	0.4	0.4
IFTA	0.8	1.1	1.9	2.4	1.8
ICell	0.9	0.9	1.3	1.8	1.3
Hyalin	1.4	1.9	2.2	2.5	2.1
IntThic	0.8	1.2	1.2	1.5	1.2

Diffuse: diffuse lesion (mesangial expansion), Nodular: nodular lesion (nodular sclerosis), SubendW: subendothelial space widening (double contour of basement membrane), Exudative: exudative lesion, MesLy: mesangiolysis/microaneurysm, PVas: peri-hilar neovascularization (polar vasculosis), GScl: global glomerulosclerosis/collapsing glomerular change · ischemic glomerular change, SScl: segmental glomerulosclerosis, GMeg: glomerulomegaly, IFTA: interstitial fibrosis and tubular atrophy, ICell: interstitial cell infiltration, Hyalin: arteriolar hyalinosis, Arterio: arteriosclerosis with intimal thickening

cases exhibited diffuse lesions. In addition, more than half of the cases exhibited IFTA, interstitial cell infiltration, arteriolar hyalinosis, and intimal thickening. These findings indicated that interstitial and vascular changes as well as glomerular change are progress even in the early clinical stage of diabetic nephropathy. Moreover, these findings indicate that progression of various pathological changes of diabetic nephropathy might be progress even before clinically confirmed diabetic nephropathy. Similar finding has been reported that pathological changes in DN can progress in patients with normal albuminuria [23]. Moreover, a high frequency of global glomerular sclerosis in normoalbuminuric and microalbuminuric patients with type 2 diabetes would participate in a loss of GFR [10]. These pathological findings are not recognized as DN in current clinical practice; therefore, pathological evaluation has not sufficiently progressed. However, an early intervention for DN should be an important step toward preventing and slowing disease progression [2]. Therefore, development of pathological change-specific biomarkers to identify the progression of diffuse, interstitial, and vascular lesions at an earlier stage is required [24].

In stage 2, more than half of the cases had polar vasculosis. This finding would be reasonable, because new generated vessels of polar vasculosis connect glomerular capillaries and peritubular capillaries. This connection might reduce the glomerular hyperfiltration of diabetic kidney in early clinical stage.

In stage 3, approximately half of the cases had subendothelial space widening, exudative lesions, nodular lesions, and mesangiolysis. These glomerular pathological changes were previously reported as typical pathological changes in diabetic

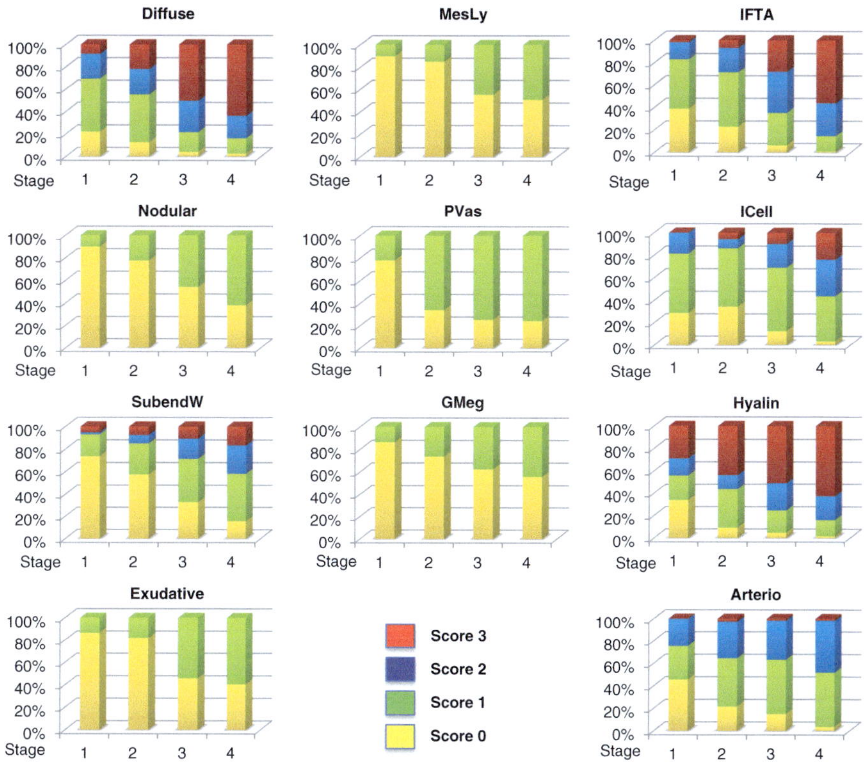

Fig. 9.1 The percent of each histological score in clinical stage of Japanese DN. Diffuse: diffuse lesion (mesangial expansion), Nodular: nodular lesion (nodular sclerosis), SubendW: subendothelial space widening (double contour of basement membrane), Exudative: exudative lesion, MesLy: mesangiolysis/microaneurysm, PVas: peri-hilar neovascularization (polar vasculosis), GMeg: glomerulomegaly, IFTA: interstitial fibrosis and tubular atrophy, ICell: interstitial cell infiltration, Hyalin: arteriolar hyalinosis, Arterio: arteriosclerosis with intimal thickening

nephropathy and reported as predictors of kidney dysfunction. It is easy to speculate that stage 3 should be good indication for kidney biopsy for diabetic cases in general condition, and these pathological findings were classically reported as a characteristic pathological changes and prognostic pathological changes. In contrast, glomerulomegaly was a minor pathological finding and reached 44% in stage 4. Each clinical stage demonstrates characteristic pathological changes.

9.8 Impacts of Pathological Findings on Clinical Outcomes

In the analysis of all 600 cases, all 13 types of pathological findings could clearly predict the occurrence of composite kidney events (dialysis, halving of eGFR, or doubling of serum Cr) (Table 9.5). This is very valuable findings. Previous many

Table 9.5 HRs for composite kidney event

	Stage 1	Stage 2	Stage 3	Stage 4	All
	Haz. Ratio	Haz. Ratio	Haz. Ratio	Haz. Ratio	Haz. Ratio
Diffuse	>500	2.1	**2.6**	3.9	**2.7**
Nodular	**35.5**	**3.9**	**1.8**	**2.0**	**2.4**
SubendW	7.5	**3.9**	**1.9**	**3.3**	**2.8**
Exudative	**35.5**	1.8	**2.1**	1.4	**2.7**
MesLy	**35.5**	**2.7**	**2.0**	1.6	**2.6**
PVas	1.1	1.4	**1.6**	1.4	**1.6**
GScl (%)	1.2	1.1	**1.1**	**1.1**	**1.2**
SScl (%)	1.0	1.7	**1.3**	**1.3**	**1.4**
GMeg	4.4	1.6	1.0	0.9	**1.3**
IFTA	0.7	2.2	**3.1**	0.3	**3.5**
ICell	0.9	2.3	**3.3**	2.8	**3.7**
Hyalin	1.2	>500	2.0	1.6	**2.3**
IntThic	1.2	2.9	1.6	2.4	**2.4**

Bold; $p < 0.05$

Diffuse: diffuse lesion (mesangial expansion), Nodular: nodular lesion (nodular sclerosis), SubendW: subendothelial space widening (double contour of basement membrane), Exudative: exudative lesion, MesLy: mesangiolysis/microaneurysm, PVas: peri-hilar neovascularization (polar vasculosis), GScl: global glomerulosclerosis/collapsing glomerular change · ischemic glomerular change, SScl: segmental glomerulosclerosis, GMeg: glomerulomegaly, IFTA: interstitial fibrosis and tubular atrophy, ICell: interstitial cell infiltration, Hyalin: arteriolar hyalinosis, Arterio: arteriosclerosis with intimal thickening

studies showed that some pathological changes, such as nodular lesions or interstitial fibrosis and tubular atrophy, were kidney prognosis predictors. However, our large number and long observation period study indicates that only limited factors were prognostic risk because of the statistical limitation due to the small number of cases. As describe in previous section, the scores of each pathological finding correlated strongly with that of other pathological findings. And, all 13 types of pathological findings could clearly predict the occurrence of composite kidney events.

After adjustments for age and gender, each pathological finding showed characteristic hazard ratios (HRs) for the composite kidney events in each clinical stage. Nodular lesions and mesangiolysis had high HRs in stages 1 and 2 (stage 1; 35.5, 35.5, stage 2; 3.9, 2.7, respectively). Exudative lesions had a high HR in stage 1 (7.5), and subendothelial space widening had a high HR in stages 2 and 4 (3.9 and 3.3, respectively). In stage 3, IFTA and interstitial cell infiltration had high HRs (3.1 and 3.3, respectively).

However, each pathological finding had different impacts on all-cause mortality. In the analysis of all cases, nodular lesions, subendothelial space widening, exudative lesions, mesangiolysis, IFTA and interstitial cell infiltration, and intimal thickening could clearly predict the occurrence of all-cause mortality (HR for each pathological finding: 2.4, 2.8, 2.1, 2.2, 2.6, 4.8, and 3.5, respectively; Table 9.6). Moreover, nodular lesions, subendothelial space widening, exudative lesions, and

Table 9.6 HRs for all-cause mortality

	Stage 1	Stage 2	Stage 3	Stage 4	All
	Haz. Ratio	Haz. Ratio	Haz. Ratio	Haz. Ratio	Haz. Ratio
Diffuse	1.0	>500	2.7	0.3	1.4
Nodular	0.0	2.0	**2.1**	1.6	**2.4**
SubendW	2.7	2.3	**2.7**	0.7	**2.8**
Exudative	0.0	3.4	**2.0**	0.5	**2.1**
MesLy	0.0	1.4	**2.7**	2.3	**2.2**
PVas	2.3	0.5	1.5	0.6	1.3
GScl (%)	1.2	0.8	1.0	1.0	1.1
SScl (%)	>500	1.1	1.2	1.2	1.1
GMeg	>500	4.6	0.6	0.6	0.7
IFTA	0.3	2.9	3.9	0.9	**2.6**
ICell	0.2	>500	4.0	0.8	**4.8**
Hyalin	1.8	**1.0**	2.1	>500	3.3
IntThic	2.0	>500	1.7	>500	**3.5**

Bold; $p < 0.05$

Diffuse: diffuse lesion (mesangial expansion), Nodular: nodular lesion (nodular sclerosis), SubendW: subendothelial space widening (double contour of basement membrane), Exudative: exudative lesion, MesLy: mesangiolysis/microaneurysm, PVas: peri-hilar neovascularization (polar vasculosis), GScl: global glomerulosclerosis/collapsing glomerular change · ischemic glomerular change, SScl: segmental glomerulosclerosis, GMeg: glomerulomegaly, IFTA: interstitial fibrosis and tubular atrophy, ICell: interstitial cell infiltration, Hyalin: arteriolar hyalinosis, Arterio: arteriosclerosis with intimal thickening

mesangiolysis had a high impact on all-cause mortality in stage 3 (HR for each pathological finding: 2.1, 2.7, 2.0, and 2.7, respectively).

The significance of pathological findings that have been reported as prognostic predictors may be affected by differences in the clinical stage. This study found that notable pathological findings progressed according to progression of clinical stages. The evaluation of adequate pathological findings at appropriate stages was effective for predicting prognosis and assessing the risk that could not be stratified by clinical stage. These results indicated that pathological findings classified the risk of kidney dysfunction and all-cause mortality in addition to the Japanese clinical classification of DN.

9.9 Summary

- Diffuse lesions were observed in many DN cases, even at the stage of normal albuminuria.
- Pathological findings such as nodular lesions and mesangiolysis were also observed in some cases at this stage. Interstitial lesions, such as interstitial cell infiltration and interstitial fibrosis or tubular atrophy, and vascular diseases, such

as arteriolar hyalinosis, arteriosclerosis, and vascular hyperplasia, are also observed in biopsy specimens of early stage diabetes cases.

- Cases with nodular lesions and mesangiolysis in the early stages had a particularly poor prognosis of kidney disease.
- It is impossible to predict the pathological findings using clinical parameters. Therefore, pathological evaluation by kidney biopsy is crucially important in clinical practice for kidney disease of diabetic patients.

9.10 Indication of Kidney Biopsy

Indication of kidney biopsy in diabetic cases is a very important issue. Although the pathological evaluation of kidney biopsy specimens for DN has various benefits, there is no clear indication for kidney biopsy so far. Particularly, in the case of normoalbuminuria or microalbuminuria, assessment of pathological findings is clinically valuable [21, 22]. However, kidney biopsy has some risks including bleeding and infection. Therefore, kidney biopsy for diabetic cases can be performed after obtaining informed consents and informing the patients of the benefits of biopsy. Cases with an atypical clinical course, such as a rapid increase of albuminuria and progressive eGFR decline, would be candidates for kidney biopsy. Accumulating the biopsy cases of diabetic patients should be considered important to verify the findings and prognosis. After accumulating knowledge of kidney biopsy value in diabetic cases, the additional discussions will be necessary to reach a consensus of kidney biopsy indication for diabetic cases.

References

1. Pavkov ME, Knowler WC, Lemley KV, Mason CC, Myers BD, Nelson RG. Early renal function decline in type 2 diabetes. Clin J Am Soc Nephrol. 2012;7(1):78–84.
2. Krolewski AS. Progressive renal decline: the new paradigm of diabetic nephropathy in type 1 diabetes. Diabetes Care. 2015;38(6):954–62.
3. Perkins BA, Ficociello LH, Ostrander BE, et al. Microalbuminuria and the risk for early progressive renal function decline in type 1 diabetes. J Am Soc Nephrol. 2007;18(4):1353–61.
4. Haneda M, Utsunomiya K, Koya D, et al. A new classification of Diabetic Nephropathy 2014: a report from Joint Committee on Diabetic Nephropathy. Clin Exp Nephrol. 2015;19(1):1–5.
5. Haneda M, Utsunomiya K, Koya D, et al. A new Classification of Diabetic Nephropathy 2014: a report from Joint Committee on Diabetic Nephropathy. J Diabetes Investig. 2015;6(2):242–6.
6. Shimizu M, Furuichi K, Toyama T, et al. Long-term outcomes of Japanese type 2 diabetic patients with biopsy-proven diabetic nephropathy. Diabetes Care. 2013;36(11):3655–62.
7. Fiorentino M, Bolignano D, Tesar V, et al. Renal biopsy in patients with diabetes: a pooled meta-analysis of 48 studies. Nephrol Dial Transplant. 2017;32(1):97–110.
8. He F, Xia X, Wu XF, Yu XQ, Huang FX. Diabetic retinopathy in predicting diabetic nephropathy in patients with type 2 diabetes and renal disease: a meta-analysis. Diabetologia. 2013;56(3):457–66.

9. Moriya T, Tanaka S, Kawasaki R, et al. Diabetic retinopathy and microalbuminuria can predict macroalbuminuria and renal function decline in Japanese type 2 diabetic patients: Japan Diabetes Complications Study. Diabetes Care. 2013;36(9):2803–9.
10. Moriya T, Suzuki Y, Inomata S, Iwano M, Kanauchi M, Haneda M. Renal histological heterogeneity and functional progress in normoalbuminuric and microalbuminuric Japanese patients with type 2 diabetes. BMJ Open Diabetes Res Care. 2014;2(1):e000029.
11. Hong D, Zheng T, Jia-qing S, Jian W, Zhi-hong L, Lei-shi L. Nodular glomerular lesion: a later stage of diabetic nephropathy? Diabetes Res Clin Pract. 2007;78(2):189–95.
12. Dalla Vestra M, Saller A, Bortoloso E, Mauer M, Fioretto P. Structural involvement in type 1 and type 2 diabetic nephropathy. Diabetes Metab. 2000;26(Suppl 4):8–14.
13. Fioretto P, Mauer M, Brocco E, et al. Patterns of renal injury in NIDDM patients with microalbuminuria. Diabetologia. 1996;39(12):1569–76.
14. Takazakura E, Nakamoto Y, Hayakawa H, Kawai K, Muramoto S. Onset and progression of diabetic glomerulosclerosis; a prospective study based on serial renal biopsies. Diabetes. 1975;24(1):1–9.
15. Shimizu M, Furuichi K, Yokoyama H, et al. Kidney lesions in diabetic patients with normoalbuminuric renal insufficiency. Clin Exp Nephrol. 2014;18(2):305–12.
16. Wada T, Haneda M, Furuichi K, et al. Clinical impact of albuminuria and glomerular filtration rate on renal and cardiovascular events, and all-cause mortality in Japanese patients with type 2 diabetes. Clin Exp Nephrol. 2014;18(4):613–20.
17. Mise K, Hoshino J, Ubara Y, et al. Renal prognosis a long time after renal biopsy on patients with diabetic nephropathy. Nephrol Dial Transplant. 2014;29(1):109–18.
18. Tervaert TW, Mooyaart AL, Amann K, et al. Pathologic classification of diabetic nephropathy. J Am Soc Nephrol. 2010;21(4):556–63.
19. An Y, Xu F, Le W, et al. Renal histologic changes and the outcome in patients with diabetic nephropathy. Nephrol Dial Transplant. 2015;30(2):257–66.
20. Manual for pathological diagnosis of diabetic nephropathy and hypertensive nephrosclerosis. Tokyo: Tokyo Igakusha; 2014.
21. Furuichi K, Yuzawa Y, Shimizu M, et al. Nationwide multicentre kidney biopsy study of Japanese patients with type 2 diabetes. Nephrol Dial Transplant. 2017;33(1):138–48.
22. Furuichi K, Shimizu M, Yuzawa Y, et al. Clinicopathological analysis of biopsy-proven diabetic nephropathy based on the Japanese classification of diabetic nephropathy. Clin Exp Nephrol. 2017;22(3):570–82.
23. Nyumura I, Honda K, Tanabe K, Teraoka S, Iwamoto Y. Early histologic lesions and risk factors for recurrence of diabetic kidney disease after kidney transplantation. Transplantation. 2012;94(6):612–9.
24. Van JA, Scholey JW, Konvalinka A. Insights into Diabetic Kidney Disease Using Urinary Proteomics and Bioinformatics. J Am Soc Nephrol. 2017;28(4):1050–61.

Part II
Pathological Aspects

Chapter 10
Evaluation of Diabetic Kidney Lesions

Junichi Hoshino

10.1 Patients Characteristics of Diabetic Nephropathy (DN): Clinical Perspectives

Clinical and pathological findings of diabetic kidney disease (DKD) are diverse. The clinical diagnosis of diabetic nephropathy (DN) in patients with diabetes mellitus usually depends on the detection of microalbuminuria (albumin excretion of more than 30 mg/g of creatinine in two out of three random urine samples collected within 6-month period) [1, 2]. A subset of diabetic patients with microalbuminuria will develop advanced DN, referred as overt nephropathy, clinical nephropathy, proteinuria, or macroalbuminuria with progressive decline in the glomerular filtration rate [2, 3]. In clinical practice, DN is often diagnosed after diagnosis of diabetic retinopathy. However, the sensitivity and specificity of diabetic retinopathy to predict diabetic nephropathy were only 0.65 (95% confidence interval (CI) 0.62, 0.68) and 0.75 (0.73, 0.78), respectively [4]. The most accurate diagnosis of DN is made by pathological evaluation of renal biopsy specimen. Nonetheless, the typical clinical indications for renal biopsy included proteinuria without diabetic retinopathy, hematuria, rapid decline in eGFR, or massive proteinuria in patients with short duration of diabetes, which is different from "typical" clinical diagnostic criteria of DN [5]. Indeed, it was reported that the prevalence of diabetic retinopathy and hematuria in a biopsy cohort was 11% and 69%, respectively [6]. Therefore as shown in the Fig. 10.1, we need to keep in mind that patient's characteristics between biopsy-proven DN cohort and DKD cohort are not identical [7].

J. Hoshino (✉)
Nephrology Center, Toranomon Hospital, Tokyo, Japan
e-mail: hoshino@toranomon.gr.jp

T. Wada et al. (eds.), *Diabetic Kidney Disease*,
https://doi.org/10.1007/978-981-15-9301-7_10

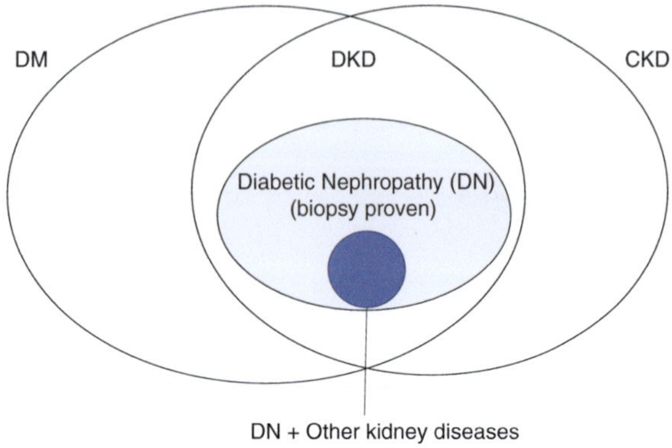

Fig. 10.1 Conceptual diagram of diabetic kidney disease, chronic kidney disease, and diabetic nephropathy (biopsy proven) [7]

10.2 Diagnosis of DN: Pathological Perspective

It is essential to evaluate renal tissue with appropriate universal standards for renal biopsy. In 1959, Gellman et al. first reported clinical correlation of renal biopsy findings [8]. Thereafter, Gambara et al. and Fioretto et al. made basic distinctions between typical and atypical DN as well as other glomerular diseases superimposed on DN [9, 10]. They defined typical DN as glomerular, tubulointerstitial, and arteriolar changes occurring in parallel. Although they are useful for research biopsies, there were some opinions that it was not practical for clinical use [11]. In 2006, the Research Committee of the Renal Pathology Society was launched and developed an international consensus classification combining type 1 and type 2 diabetic nephropathies in 2010, aiming easy to use internationally in clinical practice [11]. Their standards include hematoxylin and eosin, periodic acid-Schiff (PAS), Masson's trichrome, and periodic acid-methenamine silver stains for light microscopy. It is preferable to evaluate biopsy specimens containing at least ten glomeruli. Immunofluorescence requires the use of antibodies against IgA, IgG, IgM, C3, C1q, and kappa and lambda light chains to rule out other renal diseases. Electron microscopy must be performed as well [11]. Likewise, Wada et al. launched a Japanese nationwide study group for diabetic nephropathy with the support of the Ministry of Health, Labour and Welfare of Japan in 2009. After experience of heterogeneity of DN, including the detection of advanced DN lesions even in normoalbuminuria patients [12], they were planned to evaluate as many pathologic parameters as possible with clear definitions and standardized scores for each. Accordingly, a new pathological classification was proposed by the Japanese Renal Pathological Society (JRPS) in 2017 [5]. The details of pathological aspects of DN are also described previously (Chaps. 8 and 9).

10.3 Purposes of Renal Biopsy

In general, there are two main reasons performing renal biopsy to DKD patients—for accurate diagnosis and for outcome prediction. Because it is known that earlier intensive treatments can prevent progression of DN [13, 14], it is essential to diagnose DN accurately and start treatment earlier for better renal outcome. As described above, clinicians often choose to perform renal biopsy when patients have "atypical" clinical findings as DN, such as short duration of diabetes mellitus history (e.g., less than 5 years), without diabetic retinopathy or neuropathy, or having massive hematuria. Although the severity of diabetic retinopathy, an independent predictor for end-stage renal disease (ESRD), is highly correlated with changes in renal pathology [15], it is often difficult to suspect renal changes only from clinical features. Of 310 biopsy-proven DN patients in our hospital, 23% of them coexisted with other renal diseases except for nephrosclerosis [6]. Similar findings were reported from Colombia University. In 611 diabetic patients assessed through renal biopsy specimen in 2011, only 37% of them had "typical" diabetic nephropathy (DN) findings, with 27% of them had diagnosed coexistence of DN with nondiabetic renal disease [16]. It was reported that longer duration of diabetes (≧12 years) was associated with a greater likelihood of DN, but the sensitivity and specificity were only 58% and 73% [16]. Therefore, we should keep in mind that the pure DN could be expected just in three-quarter of the biopsy indication cohort of DN.

10.4 Pathological Changes in Early Stage of DN

It is important to know that DN pathological changes are common even in patient with early stage of DN. At earlier stage, glomerular volume is enlarged 70% as compared with the glomerular of nondiabetic subjects [17]. It was reported that in patients with type 1 diabetes with normoalbuminuric renal insufficiency, the expansion of mesangium, glomerular basement membrane (GBM) thickening, advanced arteriolar hyalinosis, and global sclerosis were prominent [18, 19]. On the other hand, in patients with type 2 diabetes with normoalbuminuric renal insufficiency, Shimizu et al. reported that diffuse lesions, nodular lesions, tubulointerstitial lesions, and vascular lesions were more advanced compared to those with preserved eGFR [12, 20]. In addition, a Japanese nationwide biopsy cohort study revealed that proportion of DN pathological changes in patients with lower-risk CKD heatmap categories (green or yellow) were, respectively, diffuse lesions, 81.6%; polar vasculosis, 42.6%; subendothelial space widening 35.1%; interstitial fibrosis and tubular atrophy (IFTA) (score ≧ 2), 21.3%; arteriolar hyalinosis (score ≧ 2), 45.7%; and arteriosclerosis (score ≧ 2), 24.2% [5]. Moreover, a recent analysis suggested these pathological changes in patients of low-risk CKD heatmap categories were associated with worse renal outcome [21], suggesting importance of early detection of pathological changes even in early clinical stage of DN. Of course, renal biopsy is a kind of invasive examination. Thus, it is inarguable the importance of careful evaluation of indication for renal biopsy. However, at this point, renal biopsy is considered as the only tool for accurate diagnosis of DN, although utility of serum or urine biomarkers has been recently reported.

10.5 Typical Pathological Findings of DN

The typical pathological findings of DN include a diffuse form with mesangial sclerosis accompanied with increase of mesangial matrix, uniform thickening of capillary walls, a nodular lesion sometimes combined with microaneurysms, and hyalinosis lesions [22]. The nodular lesion—one of the most representative findings of DN—is the type of change as first reported by Kimmelstiel and Wilson in 1936 [23], which is considered to arise from focal mesangiolysis due to mesangial and/or endothelial injury [24]. Sometimes close observation should be needed to distinguish small nodular lesion from severe diffuse lesion, since both lesions were composed of mesangial extracellular matrix. The JRPS classification defined it as a nodular expansion of mesangial extracellular matrix with loss of original capillary loop structure, while diffuse lesion remains capillary loop structure [5]. The nodular lesion is PAS-positive, green with Masson's trichrome, and black with silver stains, which is similar to the staining of diffuse lesion. However, the dyeability of PAS and PAM staining in the nodular lesion is usually weaker than that in diffuse lesion. It was reported an increase in mesangial staining for type IV and V collagen in early and moderately advanced mesangial lesions, whereas an increase only for type V and VI collagen in late nodules [25, 26], and the switch of matrix protein production might be associated with development of nodular lesions in DN [27]. PAS and PAM staining are faint at sites where type IV collagen is decreased and type VI collagen is increased in nodular lesions of human [28], and this characteristic change of collagen production—named faintly-stained nodular lesion (FASL)—was a predictor of ESRD in diabetic patients with nodular glomerulosclerosis that was independent of known indicators of renal progression [29]. The nodular lesion is also observed in membranoproliferative glomerulonephritis, amyloidosis, light-chain deposition diseases, fibrillary glomerulonephritis, immunotactoid glomerulopathy, idiopathic nodular sclerosis, etc. [30].

Mesangiolysis is an injurious glomerular process that primarily affects the mesangium. It is manifested by attenuation or dissolution of the matrix and degeneration of mesangial cells and is often observed in patients with DN [26]. Three types of mesangiolysis were proposed: (1) mesangiolysis manifested by glomerular mesangial cystic lesions, followed by features resembling proliferative glomerulonephritis, (2) mesangiolysis associated with extensive widening of the subendothelial space, and (3) mesangiolysis with lamellated mesangial nodules associated with repeated mesangial or endothelial damage [26]. It is considered as the initial lesion occurring in glomeruli in the process of diabetic nodule formation, and disturbed blood flow into glomeruli, caused by diabetic arteriosclerosis, may be implicated in the development of the mesangiolysis [28].

Hyalinosis lesion is a famous finding in glomeruli in DN as well and also called exudative lesion or "fibrin cap" [22]. This lesion is the accumulation of hyaline eosinophilic homogeneous materials between endothelial cells and the GBM of the capillary walls. However, recently "fibrin cap" is not widely used frequently because it does not contain fibrin [11, 31]. Exudative lesion in glomeruli is not a typical finding of DN, since it is often observed in other kidney diseases such as hypertensive nephrosclerosis or focal segmental glomerulosclerosis [11]. The pathogenesis of the lesion has been associated with endothelial injury and possible hemodynamic alterations [22] and could be associated with creation of mesangiolysis and nodular lesion. Therefore, subendothelial space widening in the glomeruli could be important predictor of disease progression. In addition, Stout et al. reported that insudative lesions were not only observed within the glomerular capillaries and Bowman's capsule but also in the renal arteries and the proximal convoluted tubules [32]. Recent studies of biopsy-proven DN have clearly demonstrated that glomerular and arteriolar insudative lesions show a higher frequency in patients with more advanced DN [6, 20]. Moreover, it was reported that severity of the insudative lesions of the proximal tubules—named paratubular basement membrane insudative lesions (PTBMIL)—was associated with poor renal outcome even after adjusting other factors and possible new predictor for renal outcome especially in early stage of DN [33].

Perihilar neovascularization, also known as polar vasculosis, is often an observed finding in patients with DN even in the early stage of DN [34]. In 1956, Smith et al. reported anatomical features of the human renal glomerular efferent vessel [35], and thereafter three-dimensional analysis revealed increase of vasculature around the glomerular vascular pole [36]. It is a significant, possibly hemodynamically induced, remodeling process of the glomeruli, is associated with mesangium expansion, and is suggested to serve for preservation of glomerular function [34].

Tubulointerstitial changes are also major findings of DN, described as IFTA and interstitial inflammation. The tubules were thought to show changes that reflect the degree of glomerular alterations [22]. However, as described above, severity of glomerular lesions and tubulointerstitial lesions are usually not parallel. Fioretto et al. reported that the balanced severity of glomerular, tubulointerstitial, and arteriolar changes was observed only in 30 % of patients with microalbuminuria and 50% of those with proteinuria [37], which may be influenced by the presence of cardiovascular complications and/or drug use. The presence of these lesions is not specific findings of DN. Therefore, the evaluation of tubulointerstitial disease is often comparable to other renal diseases, such as renal transplantation and nephrosclerosis [38, 39].

Arteriolar hyalinosis is a common finding in DN as well. The clinical importance in advanced DN is not large, as discussed above; however, in patients with early

DN—patients with normoalbuminuria or microalbuminuria—it is reported that index of arteriolar hyalinosis (IAH) is a possible predictor for future renal dysfunction or increase of albuminuria [40].

Most of the recent classifications, such as the RPS classification and the JRPS classification, can be detected by light microscopy, for GBM thickening that is confirmed by electron microscopy. On the other hand, the occurrence of linear immunofluorescent staining for immunoglobulin G along the glomerular capillary walls is a typical finding of DN, too. The mechanism of this staining has not been clarified, but it is considered that the main mechanism of linear IgG staining in DN could be penetration of serum proteins into the basement membrane secondary to charge and size selectivity impairment with consequent GBM thickening [41–43]. Westberg et al. concluded that the consistent presence of albumin and the frequent absence of complement components at the sites of staining provided evidence against an immunologic mechanism for this immunofluorescent staining [41]. Another hypothesis of the mechanism for the IgG staining is formation of immune complexes between insulin and anti-insulin antibodies [44, 45]. Importantly, more intense linear immunoglobulin G staining is associated with worse renal outcome after adjusting possible clinical and pathological confounders [46].

10.6 Evaluation of DN by RPS and JRPS

The RPS classification published in 2010 is based on glomerular lesions, with a separate evaluation for interstitial and vascular lesions [11]. The glomerular scores were classified as follows: class I, glomerular basement membrane thickening (>395 nm in females, >430 nm in males) by EM without any of the other glomerular criteria detailed below for classes II, III, and IV; class IIa, mild mesangial expansion (the expanded mesangial area is smaller than the mean area of capillary lumen) in >25% of the observed mesangial areas; class IIb, severe mesangial expansion (the expanded mesangial area is larger than the mean area of capillary lumen) in >25% of the total observed mesangial areas; class III, nodular sclerosis known as Kimmelstiel-Wilson lesion and <50% global glomerulosclerosis; and class IV, >50% global glomerulosclerosis. The IFTA scores were classified as follows: 0, absent; 1 (mild), <25%; 2 (moderate), 25–50%; and 3 (severe), >50% of the total area. Interstitial inflammation was scored as follows: 0, absent; 1 (mild), inflammation related only to IFTA; and 2 (advanced), inflammation in areas without IFTA. Arteriolar hyalinosis was scored as follows: 0, absent; 1 (mild), hyalinosis of, at least, one arteriole; and 2 (advanced), hyalinosis of more than one arteriole. Arteriosclerosis was scored in the most severely affected artery as follows: 0, no intimal thickening; 1 (mild), intimal thickening that was less than the medial thickness; and 2 (advanced), intimal thickening that was greater than the medial thickness (Table 10.1).

On the other hand, the JRPS classification, published in 2017, is evaluated based on nine glomerular lesions, two interstitial lesions, and two vascular lesions [5]. The

Table 10.1 Comparison of pathological evaluation by RPS and JRPS

Pathological findings	RPS (score)	Definition of score	JRPS (score)	Definition of score
Glomerular lesions	Class I Nonspecific change in LM	GBM > 395 nm in female GBM > 430 nm in male	[a]Diffuse lesion (mesangial expansion) (0–3)	0 normal or mild mesangial expansion 1 mesangial expansion ≦ capillary lumen 2 mesangial expansion = capillary lumen 3 mesangial expansion ≧ capillary lumen
	Class IIa Mild mesangial expansion	Mild mesangial expansion in >25% of the observed mesangium	Nodular lesion (0/1)	0 (note detected), 1 (detected)
			[b]Subendothelial space widening (double contour of basement membrane) (0–3)	Double contour basement membrane (%) (determined in peripheral capillary of the most severe glomerulus) 0 (<10%), 1 (10–25%), 2 (25–50%), 3 (≧50%)
	Class IIb Severe mesangial expansion	Severe mesangial expansion in >25% of the observed mesangium	Exudative lesion (0/1)	0 (not detected), 1 (detected)
			[b]Polar vasculosis (0/1)	0 (not detected), 1 (detected)
			Global glomerulosclerosis (%)	Number of glomerulosclerosis/all glomeruli
	Class III Nodular sclerosis	Nodular sclerosis	Segmental glomerulosclerosis (%)	Number of glomerulosclerosis/all glomeruli
	Class IV Advanced diabetic glomerulosclerosis	Global glomerular sclerosis in >50% of glomeruli	[b]Glomerulomegaly (0/1)	Glomeruli >250 μm in diameter 0 (not detected), 1 (detected)
Interstitial lesions	Interstitial fibrosis and tubular atrophy (IFTA) (0–3)	0 (no IFTA), 1 (<25%), 2 (25–50%), 3 (≧50%)	Interstitial fibrosis and tubular atrophy (IFTA) (0–3)	Same as RPS
	Interstitial inflammation (0–2)	0 (absent), 1 (infiltration only in relation to IFTA), 2 (infiltration in areas without IFTA)	[a]Interstitial inflammation (0–3)	0 (no cell infiltration), 1 (<25%), 2 (25–50%), 3 (≧50%)

(continued)

Table 10.1 (continued)

Pathological findings	RPS (score)	Definition of score	JRPS (score)	Definition of score
Vascular lesions	Arteriolar hyalinosis (0–2)	0 (absent), 1 (at least one area of arteriolar hyalinosis), 2 (>1 area of arteriolar hyalinosis)	[a]Arteriolar hyalinosis (0–3)	0 (no hyalinosis), 1 (one or more partial arteriolar hyalinosis), 2 (approximately 50% hyalinosis), 3 (more than 50% hyalinosis, or penetrating hyalinosis)
	Intimal thickening (0–2)	0 (no intimal thickening), 1 (intimal thickness/media thickness < 1), 2 (intimal thickening and intimal thickness/media thickness ≧ 1)	Intimal thickening (0–2)	Same as RPS

[a]More detailed definition in the JRPS classification than those in the RPS classification
[b]Newly proposed definitions in the JRPS classification

nine glomerular lesions comprised a diffuse lesion (score 0–3), nodular lesion (score 0/1), subendothelial space widening or duplication of the basement membrane (subendothelial widening) (score 0–3), exudative lesion (score 0/1), mesangiolysis (microaneurysm) (score 0/1), polar vasculosis (or perihilar neovascularization) (score 0/1), global glomerulosclerosis/collapsing glomerular change and ischemic glomerular change (%), segmental glomerulosclerosis (%), and glomerulomegaly (score 0/1). There is a slight change in the interstitial lesions and vascular lesions, with four classes of evaluation of interstitial inflammation score and arteriolar hyalinosis (0–3), while 3 classes of evaluations in RPS classification. The evaluation system in IFTA and intimal thickening was identical in both classifications. In short, compared to RPS classification, this classification comprises four new more detailed pathological features, subendothelial widening, polar vasculosis, mesangiolysis, and glomerulomegaly, as well as three other features increasing the number of grade from 3 to 4 in mesangial expansion, interstitial inflammation, and arteriolar hyalinosis. And recent study suggested that presence of polar vasculosis and/or subendothelial space widening, which are newly proposed by the JRPS classification, should be important findings for diagnosis of DN [5].

10.7 Renal Biopsy Findings and Renal Prognosis

The second reason for renal biopsy is a prognostic purpose. After establishment of the pathological classification by RPS and JRPS, the next question should be who needs to be treated and how. In order to clarify the impact of each pathological

Table 10.2 The RPS pathological scoring system (D-score)

Variables	Grade	Score	Variables	Grade	Score
Glomerular	I	0	Interstitial inflammation	0	0
	IIa	3		1	3
	IIb	4		2	4
	III, IV	6	Hyalinosis	0, 1	0
IFTA	0	0		2	3
	1	7	Arteriosclerosis	0, 1	0
	2	9		2	1
	3	11	Total		25

Table 10.3 The JRPS pathological scoring system (J-score)

Variables	Grade	Score	Variables	Grade	Score
Diffuse	0, 1	0	Interstitial inflammation	0	0
	2, 3	1		1, 2	5
Double	0–2	0		3	4
	3	2	Hyalinosis	0	0
Mesangiolysis		4		1–3	2
Polar vasculosis		1	Total		19
IFTA	1	0			
	2	3			
	3, 4	4			

change on renal outcome, new pathological scoring systems for predicting renal outcome by using RPS and JRPS classifications were proposed [21, 47] (Tables 10.2 and 10.3). Although it is unknown whether these scores are useful in other DN biopsy cohorts, it was reported that prediction of DN patients' renal outcome was better with either the D-scores by RPS classification or the J-scores by JRPS classification than without it. And the expected renal outcomes were >18 years in patients with J-score 0–5, 12.5 (interquartile range, 4.8, 22.3) years in those with J-score 6–10, 4.0 (1.9, 9.9) years in those with J-score 11–15, and 1.7 (1.0, 2.4) years in those with J-score 16–19, respectively (Figs. 10.2 and 10.3). Importantly, both scoring systems have higher scores in tubulointerstitial lesions compared to scores in glomerular lesions. The highest score of glomerular lesion was 6, whereas that of IFTA was 11 in the D-score and that of glomerular lesion was 4, whereas those of IFTA and interstitial inflammation were 4 and 5 in the J-score. These data suggest that, even after adjustment for urinary protein and other confounders, IFTA and interstitial inflammation are stronger factors associated with worse renal outcome than glomerular lesions, which need to be focused on. Recently, the importance of tubulointerstitial lesions was reported not only in patients with DN but also those with other renal diseases [48–51]. In addition, diabetic patients with "atypical" DN are increasing in the modern era, having mild changes in glomerulus but severe changes in tubulointerstitial lesions [52]. And as a result, crude renal outcome in the modern era was not dramatically improved from that of the older era (unpublished data). Therefore, it is desirable to find more accurate biomarkers of tubulointerstitial injury and inflammation. A study from the Joslin Diabetes Center

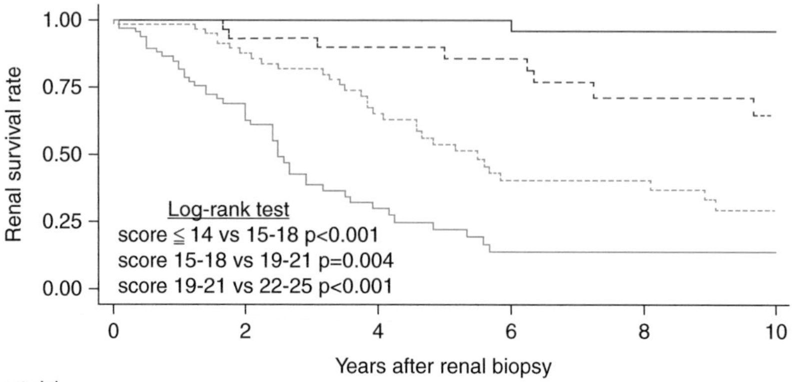

Number at risk

	0	2	4	6	8	10
D-score ≦ 14	33	29	27	26	24	21
D-score 15-18	32	29	25	19	11	10
D-score 19-21	70	47	29	15	12	8
D-score 22-25	70	36	13	5	3	1

D-score ≦ 14 — D-score 15-18 — D-score 19-21 — D-score 22-25

Fig. 10.2 Renal survival after renal biopsy dividing by D-score categories

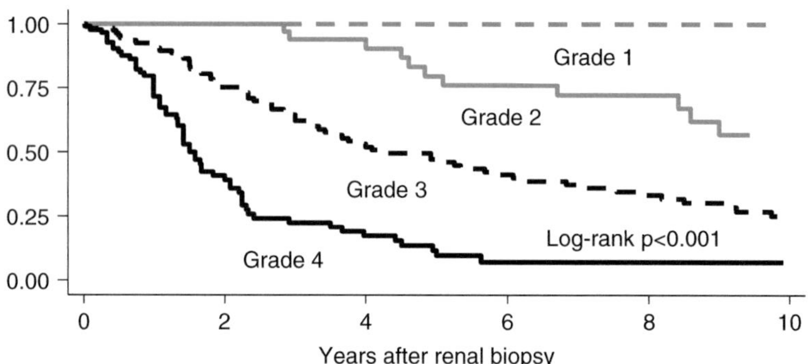

Number at risk

	0	2	4	6	8	10
Grade 1	23	20	20	19	18	16
Grade 2	39	36	27	20	15	10
Grade 3	120	71	46	33	23	12
Grade 4	89	25	10	3	3	1

Grade 1, J-score 0-5
Grade 2, J-score 6-10
Grade 3, J-score 11-15
Grade 4, J-score 16-19

Fig. 10.3 Renal survival after renal biopsy dividing by J-score categories. Grade 1, J-score 0–5. Grade 2, J-score 6–10. Grade 3, J-score 11–15. Grade 4, J-score 16–19

showed that urinary NAG and kidney injury molecule 1 (KIM-1) were markers of renal tubular injury that could predict regression of microalbuminuria in patients with type 1 diabetes [53]. Clinical utility for prediction of renal prognosis in patients with type 2 diabetes by serum levels of tumor necrosis factor-alpha (TNFα) receptors 1 and 2, the urinary concentrations of neutrophil gelatinase-associated lipocalin (NGAL), and liver fatty acid-binding protein (L-FABP) were reported as well [54–56]. Although urinary-NAG excretion was significantly correlated with the severity of tubulointerstitial injury, there was a distinct difference of predictive power between actual tubulointerstitial injury and the urinary marker. It was reported that the IFTA score was a better predictive marker for renal prognosis than urinary-NAG excretion [50]. It is still a big challenging problem in front of us to treat these tubulointerstitial lesions. In addition, the J-score system suggested the importance of the presence of mesangiolysis, which is a new glomerular parameter proposed by JRPS, for prediction of worse renal outcome [21]. Evaluation of mesangiolysis, which is newly proposed by the JRPS classification, should be important for prediction of renal outcome and/or assessment of drug efficacy.

In addition, pathological information may have some advantage for prediction of renal outcome, regardless of scoring systems for RPS and JRPS [21, 47], though improvement of clinical prediction system and/or utility of serum/urinary biomarkers may minimize the possible advantage in the near future. With recent advance in modern epidemiology, clinical prediction models themselves are improving their prediction ability, too. In 2011, Tangri et al. created the Kidney Failure Risk Equation (KFRE) for predicting risk of ESRD in patients with CKD stages 3–5, using Cox proportional hazards regression models [57]. The KFRE with only four clinical variables (age, gender, eGFR, and urinary albumin-to-creatinine ratio) predicted those at high risk of ESRD with excellent performance (KFRE index = (age/10) * ln(0.84) + gender * ln(0.93) + (eGFR/5) * ln(0.80) + ln(ACR) * ln(1.17)) [57, 58]. However, evaluation of pathological lesions of DN is still essential for accurate diagnosis, choice of the treatment, outcome prediction, and improving understanding of the mechanism of the disease.

References

1. American Diabetes Association. Standards of medical care in diabetes 2013. Diabetes Care. 2013;36(Suppl 1):S11–66.
2. Gonzalez Suarez ML, Thomas DB, Barisoni L, Fornoni A. Diabetic nephropathy: is it time yet for routine kidney biopsy? World J Diabetes. 2013;4:245–55.
3. Tang SCW, Chan GCW, Lai KN. Recent advances in managing and understanding diabetic nephropathy. F1000Research. 2016;5:F1000 Faculty Rev-1044.
4. He F, Xia X, Wu XF, Yu XQ, Huang FX. Diabetic retinopathy in predicting diabetic nephropathy in patients with type 2 diabetes and renal disease: a meta-analysis. Diabetologia. 2013;56:457–66.
5. Furuichi K, Yuzawa Y, Shimizu M, Hara A, Toyama T, Kitamura H, Suzuki Y, Sato H, Uesugi N, Ubara Y, Hisano S, Ueda Y, Nishi S, Yokoyama H, Nishino T, Kohagura K, Ogawa D, Mise K, Shibagaki Y, Kimura K, Haneda M, Makino H, Matsuo S, Wada T. Nationwide multicen-

tre kidney biopsy study of Japanese patients with type 2 diabetes. Nephrol Dial Transplant. 2017;33(1):138–48.
6. Mise K, Hoshino J, Ubara Y, Sumida K, Hiramatsu R, Hasegawa E, Yamanouchi M, Hayami N, Suwabe T, Sawa N, Fujii T, Ohashi K, Hara S, Takaichi K. Renal prognosis a long time after renal biopsy on patients with diabetic nephropathy. Nephrol Dial Transplant. 2014;29:109–18.
7. Mise K, Hoshino J. The significance of renal biopsy in diabetic kidney disease [Japanese]. Diabetes. Tokyo, Igaku Shuppan. 2017. p. 25–31.
8. Gellman DD, Pirani CL, Soothill JF, Muehrcke RC, Kark RM. Diabetic nephropathy: a clinical and pathologic study based on renal biopsies. Medicine. 1959;38:321–67.
9. Gambara V, Mecca G, Remuzzi G, Bertani T. Heterogeneous nature of renal lesions in type II diabetes. J Am Soc Nephrol. 1993;3:1458–66.
10. Fioretto P, Mauer M, Brocco E, Velussi M, Frigato F, Muollo B, Sambataro M, Abaterusso C, Baggio B, Crepaldi G, Nosadini R. Patterns of renal injury in NIDDM patients with microalbuminuria. Diabetologia. 1996;39:1569–76.
11. Tervaert TW, Mooyaart AL, Amann K, Cohen AH, Cook HT, Drachenberg CB, Ferrario F, Fogo AB, Haas M, de Heer E, Joh K, Noel LH, Radhakrishnan J, Seshan SV, Bajema IM, Bruijn JA. Pathologic classification of diabetic nephropathy. J Am Soc Nephrol. 2010;21:556–63.
12. Shimizu M, Furuichi K, Yokoyama H, Toyama T, Iwata Y, Sakai N, Kaneko S, Wada T. Kidney lesions in diabetic patients with normoalbuminuric renal insufficiency. Clin Exp Nephrol. 2014;18:305–12.
13. Fioretto P, Steffes MW, Sutherland DE, Goetz FC, Mauer M. Reversal of lesions of diabetic nephropathy after pancreas transplantation. N Engl J Med. 1998;339:69–75.
14. Makino H, Haneda M, Babazono T, Moriya T, Ito S, Iwamoto Y, Kawamori R, Takeuchi M, Katayama S. Microalbuminuria reduction with telmisartan in normotensive and hypertensive Japanese patients with type 2 diabetes: a post-hoc analysis of The Incipient to Overt: Angiotensin II Blocker, Telmisartan, Investigation on Type 2 Diabetic Nephropathy (INNOVATION) study. Hypertens Res. 2008;31:657–64.
15. Yamanouchi M, Mori M, Hoshino J, Kinowaki K, Fujii T, Ohashi K, Furuichi K, Wada T, Ubara Y. Retinopathy progression and the risk of end-stage kidney disease: results from a longitudinal Japanese cohort of 232 patients with type 2 diabetes and biopsy-proven diabetic kidney disease. BMJ Open Diabetes Res Care. 2019;7:e000726.
16. Sharma SG, Bomback AS, Radhakrishnan J, Herlitz LC, Stokes MB, Markowitz GS, D'Agati VD. The modern spectrum of renal biopsy findings in patients with diabetes. Clin J Am Soc Nephrol. 2013;8:1718–24.
17. Osterby R. Structural changes in the diabetic kidney. Clin Endocrinol Metab. 1986;15:733–51.
18. Lane PH, Steffes MW, Mauer SM. Glomerular structure in IDDM women with low glomerular filtration rate and normal urinary albumin excretion. Diabetes. 1992;41:581–6.
19. Caramori ML, Fioretto P, Mauer M. Low glomerular filtration rate in normoalbuminuric type 1 diabetic patients: an indicator of more advanced glomerular lesions. Diabetes. 2003;52:1036–40.
20. Shimizu M, Furuichi K, Toyama T, Kitajima S, Hara A, Kitagawa K, Iwata Y, Sakai N, Takamura T, Yoshimura M, Yokoyama H, Kaneko S, Wada T. Long-term outcomes of Japanese type 2 diabetic patients with biopsy-proven diabetic nephropathy. Diabetes Care. 2013;36:3655–62.
21. Hoshino J, Furuichi K, Yamanouchi M, Mise K, Kawada M, Sumida K, Hiramatsu R, Hasegawa E, Hayami N, Suwabe T, Sawa N, Hara S, Fujii T, Ohashi K, Kitagawa K, Toyama T, Shimizu M, Takaichi K, Ubara Y, Wada T. A new pathological scoring system by the Japanese classification to predict renal outcome in diabetic nephropathy. PLoS One. 2017;13(2):e0190923.
22. Jennette JC, Olson JL, Schwartz MM, Silva FG, editors. Heptinstall's pathology of the kidney. Philadelphia: Lippincott Williams & Wilkins.
23. Kimmelstiel P, Wilson C. Intercapillary lesions in the glomeruli of the kidney. Am J Pathol. 1936;12:83–98.87.
24. Silbiger S, Crowley S, Shan Z, Brownlee M, Satriano J, Schlondorff D. Nonenzymatic glycation of mesangial matrix and prolonged exposure of mesangial matrix to elevated glucose reduces collagen synthesis and proteoglycan charge. Kidney Int. 1993;43:853–64.

25. Paueksakon P, Revelo MP, Ma LJ, Marcantoni C, Fogo AB. Microangiopathic injury and augmented PAI-1 in human diabetic nephropathy. Kidney Int. 2002;61:2142–8.
26. Morita T, Yamamoto T, Churg J. Mesangiolysis: an update. Am J Kidney Dis. 1998;31:559–73.
27. Nerlich AG, Schleicher ED, Wiest I, Specks U, Timpl R. Immunohistochemical localization of collagen VI in diabetic glomeruli. Kidney Int. 1994;45:1648–56.
28. Wada T, Shimizu M, Yokoyama H, Iwata Y, Sakai Y, Kaneko S, Furuichi K. Nodular lesions and mesangiolysis in diabetic nephropathy. Clin Exp Nephrol. 2013;17:3–9.
29. Mise K, Ueno T, Hoshino J, Hazue R, Sumida K, Yamanouchi M, Hayami N, Suwabe T, Hiramatsu R, Hasegawa E, Sawa N, Fujii T, Hara S, Wada J, Makino H, Takaichi K, Ohashi K, Ubara Y. Nodular lesions in diabetic nephropathy: collagen staining and renal prognosis. Diabetes Res Clin Pract. 2017;127:187–97.
30. Raparia K, Usman I, Kanwar YS. Renal morphologic lesions reminiscent of diabetic nephropathy. Arch Pathol Lab Med. 2013;137:351–9.
31. Najafian B, Alpers CE, Fogo AB. Pathology of human diabetic nephropathy. Contrib Nephrol. 2011;170:36–47.
32. Stout LC, Kumar S, Whorton EB. Insudative lesions—their pathogenesis and association with glomerular obsolescence in diabetes: a dynamic hypothesis based on single views of advancing human diabetic nephropathy. Hum Pathol. 1994;25:1213–27.
33. Mise K, Yamaguchi Y, Hoshino J, Ueno T, Sekine A, Sumida K, Yamanouchi M, Hayami N, Suwabe T, Hiramatsu R, Hasegawa E, Sawa N, Fujii T, Hara S, Sugiyama H, Makino H, Wada J, Ohashi K, Takaichi K, Ubara Y. Paratubular basement membrane insudative lesions predict renal prognosis in patients with type 2 diabetes and biopsy-proven diabetic nephropathy. PLoS One. 2017;12:e0183190.
34. Stout LC, Whorton EB. Pathogenesis of extra efferent vessel development in diabetic glomeruli. Hum Pathol. 2007;38:1167–77.
35. Smith JP. Anatomical features of the human renal glomerular efferent vessel. J Anat. 1956;90:290–2.
36. Min W, Yamanaka N. Three-dimensional analysis of increased vasculature around the glomerular vascular pole in diabetic nephropathy. Virchows Archiv A Pathol Anat Histopathol. 1993;423:201–7.
37. Fioretto P, Mauer M. Histopathology of diabetic nephropathy. Semin Nephrol. 2007;27:195–207.
38. Solez K, Colvin RB, Racusen LC, Sis B, Halloran PF, Birk PE, Campbell PM, Cascalho M, Collins AB, Demetris AJ, Drachenberg CB, Gibson IW, Grimm PC, Haas M, Lerut E, Liapis H, Mannon RB, Marcus PB, Mengel M, Mihatsch MJ, Nankivell BJ, Nickeleit V, Papadimitriou JC, Platt JL, Randhawa P, Roberts I, Salinas-Madriga L, Salomon DR, Seron D, Sheaff M, Weening JJ. Banff'05 Meeting Report: differential diagnosis of chronic allograft injury and elimination of chronic allograft nephropathy ('CAN'). Am J Transplant. 2007;7:518–26.
39. [Manual for pathological diagnosis of diabetic nephropathy and hypertensive nephrosclerosis]. Nihon Jinzo Gakkai Shi. 2015;57:649–725.
40. Moriya T, Omura K, Matsubara M, Yoshida Y, Hayama K, Ouchi M. Arteriolar hyalinosis Predicts increase in albuminuria and GFR decline in normo- and microalbuminuric Japanese patients with type 2 diabetes. Diabetes Care. 2017;40:1373–8.
41. Westberg NG, Michael AF. Immunohistopathology of diabetic glomerulosclerosis. Diabetes. 1972;21:163–74.
42. Ainsworth SK, Hirsch HZ, Brackett NC Jr, Brissie RM, Williams AV Jr, Hennigar GR. Diabetic glomerulonephropathy: histopathologic, immunofluorescent, and ultrastructural studies of 16 cases. Hum Pathol. 1982;13:470–8.
43. Miller K, Michael AF. Immunopathology of renal extracellular membranes in diabetes mellitus. Specificity of tubular basement-membrane immunofluorescence. Diabetes. 1976;25:701–8.
44. Berns AW, Hirata Y, Blumenthal HT. Application of fluorescence microscopy to the study of possible insulin-binding reactions in formalin-fixed material. J Lab Clin Med. 1962;60:535–51.
45. Farrant PC, Shedden WI. Observations on the uptake of insulin conjugated with fluorescein isothiocyanate by diabetic kidney tissue. Diabetes. 1965;14:274–8.

46. Mise K, Hoshino J, Ueno T, Sumida K, Hiramatsu R, Hasegawa E, Yamanouchi M, Hayami N, Suwabe T, Sawa N, Fujii T, Hara S, Ohashi K, Takaichi K, Ubara Y. Clinical implications of linear immunofluorescent staining for immunoglobulin G in patients with diabetic nephropathy. Diabetes Res Clin Pract. 2014;106:522–30.
47. Hoshino J, Mise K, Ueno T, Imafuku A, Kawada M, Sumida K, Hiramatsu R, Hasegawa E, Yamanouchi M, Hayami N, Suwabe T, Sawa N, Hara S, Fujii T, Ohashi K, Ubara Y, Takaichi K. A pathological scoring system to predict renal outcome in diabetic nephropathy. Am J Nephrol. 2015;41:337–44.
48. Alamartine E, Sauron C, Laurent B, Sury A, Seffert A, Mariat C. The use of the Oxford classification of IgA nephropathy to predict renal survival. Clin J Am Soc Nephrol. 2011;6:2384–8.
49. Hsieh C, Chang A, Brandt D, Guttikonda R, Utset TO, Clark MR. Predicting outcomes of lupus nephritis with tubulointerstitial inflammation and scarring. Arthritis Care Res (Hoboken). 2011;63:865–74.
50. Mise K, Hoshino J, Ueno T, Hazue R, Hasegawa J, Sekine A, Sumida K, Hiramatsu R, Hasegawa E, Yamanouchi M, Hayami N, Suwabe T, Sawa N, Fujii T, Hara S, Ohashi K, Takaichi K, Ubara Y. Prognostic value of tubulointerstitial lesions, urinary n-acetyl-beta-d-glucosaminidase, and urinary beta2-microglobulin in patients with type 2 diabetes and biopsy-proven diabetic nephropathy. Clin J Am Soc Nephrol. 2016;11:593–601.
51. Yamanouchi M, Hoshino J, Ubara Y, Takaichi K, Kinowaki K, Fujii T, Ohashi K, Mise K, Toyama T, Hara A, Shimizu M, Furuichi K, Wada T. Clinicopathological predictors for progression of chronic kidney disease in nephrosclerosis: a biopsy-based cohort study. Nephrol Dial Transplant. 2019;34:1182–8.
52. Yamanouchi M, Furuichi K, Hoshino J, Toyama T, Hara A, Shimizu M, Kinowaki K, Fujii T, Ohashi K, Yuzawa Y, Kitamura H, Suzuki Y, Sato H, Uesugi N, Hisano S, Ueda Y, Nishi S, Yokoyama H, Nishino T, Samejima K, Kohagura K, Shibagaki Y, Mise K, Makino H, Matsuo S, Ubara Y, Wada T. Nonproteinuric versus proteinuric phenotypes in diabetic kidney disease: a propensity score-matched analysis of a nationwide, biopsy-based cohort study. Diabetes Care. 2019;42(5):891–902.
53. Vaidya VS, Niewczas MA, Ficociello LH, Johnson AC, Collings FB, Warram JH, Krolewski AS, Bonventre JV. Regression of microalbuminuria in type 1 diabetes is associated with lower levels of urinary tubular injury biomarkers, kidney injury molecule-1, and N-acetyl-beta-D-glucosaminidase. Kidney Int. 2011;79:464–70.
54. Fufaa GD, Weil EJ, Nelson RG, Hanson RL, Bonventre JV, Sabbisetti V, Waikar SS, Mifflin TE, Zhang X, Xie D, Hsu CY, Feldman HI, Coresh J, Vasan RS, Kimmel PL, Liu KD. Association of urinary KIM-1, L-FABP, NAG and NGAL with incident end-stage renal disease and mortality in American Indians with type 2 diabetes mellitus. Diabetologia. 2015;58:188–98.
55. Niewczas MA, Gohda T, Skupien J, Smiles AM, Walker WH, Rosetti F, Cullere X, Eckfeldt JH, Doria A, Mayadas TN, Warram JH, Krolewski AS. Circulating TNF receptors 1 and 2 predict ESRD in type 2 diabetes. J Am Soc Nephrol. 2012;23:507–15.
56. Pavkov ME, Nelson RG, Knowler WC, Cheng Y, Krolewski AS, Niewczas MA. Elevation of circulating TNF receptors 1 and 2 increases the risk of end-stage renal disease in American Indians with type 2 diabetes. Kidney Int. 2015;87:812–9.
57. Tangri N, Stevens LA, Griffith J, Tighiouart H, Djurdjev O, Naimark D, Levin A, Levey AS. A predictive model for progression of chronic kidney disease to kidney failure. JAMA. 2011;305:1553–9.
58. Tangri N, Grams ME, Levey AS, Coresh J, Appel LJ, Astor BC, Chodick G, Collins AJ, Djurdjev O, Elley CR, Evans M, Garg AX, Hallan SI, Inker LA, Ito S, Jee SH, Kovesdy CP, Kronenberg F, Heerspink HJ, Marks A, Nadkarni GN, Navaneethan SD, Nelson RG, Titze S, Sarnak MJ, Stengel B, Woodward M, Iseki K. Multinational assessment of accuracy of equations for predicting risk of kidney failure: a meta-analysis. JAMA. 2016;315:164–74.

Chapter 11
Nephrosclerosis and Diabetic Kidney Disease

Masayuki Yamanouchi, Kengo Furuichi, and Takashi Wada

11.1 Nephrosclerosis

People with nephrosclerosis are one of the fastest growing demographic groups in all developed countries and many developing countries as a consequence of the increasing number of elderly people as well as those with hyperglycemia, hypertension, obesity, and/or dyslipidemia [1]. Nephrosclerosis is now a major cause of ESRD, along with diabetic kidney disease and glomerulonephritis, in the USA, Europe, and Japan [2–4]. Despite attracting more attention recently, nephrosclerosis remains poorly understood, especially with regard to its pathological features and their association with progression of CKD [5–7]. This is mostly because there is a lack of kidney biopsy data from people with suspected nephrosclerosis, who are older and have hyperglycemia, hypertension, obesity, and/or dyslipidemia. Nephrosclerosis is defined pathologically by an increase of segmental or global sclerosis, interstitial fibrosis, tubular atrophy, and arteriosclerosis [8], although it has also been diagnosed clinically on the basis of albuminuria and renal impairment in older persons and patients with chronic lifestyle-related diseases. However, even data on the influence of clinical features on the renal prognosis in patients with nephrosclerosis are limited and inconsistent [9–15]. Most studies have shown that albuminuria and a decline of the glomerular filtration rate are independent risk factors for ESRD in people with nephrosclerosis, but the results for other clinical factors (age, gender, race, hyperuricemia, serum albumin, hemoglobin, BMI, and

M. Yamanouchi (✉)
Nephrology Center, Toranomon Hospital, Tokyo, Japan
e-mail: m.yamanouchi@toranomon.gr.jp

K. Furuichi
Department of Nephrology, Kanazawa Medical University School of Medicine, Ishikawa, Japan

T. Wada
Department of Nephrology and Laboratory Medicine, Kanazawa University, Ishikawa, Japan

T. Wada et al. (eds.), *Diabetic Kidney Disease*,
https://doi.org/10.1007/978-981-15-9301-7_11

systolic blood pressure) have been inconsistent. Again, this is possibly due to the limited number of biopsy-based studies on nephrosclerosis, since many patients with a clinical diagnosis of nephrosclerosis may actually have a different kidney disease or a concomitant kidney disease.

Against this background, the present study was performed with two objectives: (1) to examine clinicopathological features in patients with biopsy-proven nephrosclerosis and (2) to assess the association these features with CKD progression.

This is a retrospective study of 184 patients who underwent clinical, renal biopsy performed in 13 centers across Japan and had a pathological diagnosis of nephrosclerosis [16]. Table 11.1 shows the clinical characteristics of the study group at the time of biopsy corresponding to CKD heat map categorization [17], in which patients with CKD were categorized into four groups: green, low risk; yellow, moderately increased risk; orange, high risk; and red, very high risk. Owing to the limited number of cases, the green and yellow groups were combined into one group (G&Y) for the purposes of this study. The mean age was 55.5 ± 12.0 years, and 66% of the patients were male. The mean BP was 139.6 ± 21.2/83.9 ± 16.9 mmHg. Age was significantly higher and BMI was lower in the red group compared with the orange group. In contrast, gender, systolic BP, diastolic BP, total cholesterol, urinary occult blood, usage of RAS, CCB, and lipid-lowering drugs exhibited no significant differences among the groups.

Pathological features were also evaluated according to the following criteria.

Global Glomerulosclerosis/Collapsing Glomerular Change and Ischemic Glomerular Change (GScle) All capillaries are sclerosed, the capillary lumen is not detected, and the capillaries are collapsing.

Table 11.1 Clinical characteristics of the study group at the time of biopsy corresponding to CKD heat map categorization

Heat map	Green & Yellow ($n = 36$)	Orange ($n = 57$)	Red ($n = 91$)	Total ($n = 184$)
Age (years old)	53.17 ± 12.86	53.60 ± 10.84	57.62 ± 12.18**	55.50 ± 12.04
Gender (Male)	61%	70%	56%	66%
BMI	26.05 ± 3.56	26.61 ± 9.21	24.22 ± 3.65**	25.31 ± 6.01
SysBP (mmHg)	142.30 ± 16.22	134.95 ± 16.07	141.65 ± 25.21	139.59 ± 21.18
DiaBP (mmHg)	81.55 ± 9.89	81.58 ± 12.42	86.37 ± 21.08	83.89 ± 16.94
Cr (mg/dL)	0.82 ± 0.21	0.94 ± 0.24	1.69 ± 1.03*	1.29 ± 0.84
Tcho (mg/dL)	234.44 ± 183.23	220.85 ± 146.62	213.64 ± 48.71	220.33 ± 122.23
Ualb (g/day)	0.13 ± 0.08	0.93 ± 3.54	0.76 ± 1.05	0.69 ± 2.13
UOB	0.00, 0.00–0.50	0.00, 0.00–1.00	0.00, 0.00–0.50	0.00, 0.00–0.50
RAS	37%	37%	47%	42%
CCB	34%	46%	49%	45%
LipidDrg	9%	19%	24%	20%

BMI body mass index, *sysBP* systolic blood pressure, *diaBP* diastolic blood pressure, *Cr* creatinine, *Tcho* total cholesterol, *UAlb* urinary levels of albumin, *UOB* occult blood in urine (UOB was converted into scores as follows: (−) to 0, (±) to 0.5, (1+) to 1, (2+) to 2, and (3+) to 3), RAS: use of renin-angiotensin system inhibitor, CCB: use of calcium channel blocker, LipidDrug: use of lipid-lowering drug

*$p < 0.05$ to G&Y, and orange, **$p < 0.05$ to orange, mean ± SD or median, IQR [16]

Segmental Glomerulosclerosis (SSCle) In segmental glomerulosclerosis, a portion of the glomerulocapillaries is sclerosed.

Glomerulomegaly (GMeg) In glomerulomegaly, the diameter of one or more glomerulus in all biopsy specimens is more than 250 lm.

Interstitial Fibrosis and Tubular Atrophy (IFTA) Interstitial fibrosis is defined by the accumulation of collagen and related molecules in the interstitium. Tubular atrophy is defined by a decrease in tubular diameter and number.

Interstitial Cell Infiltration (ICell) Inflammatory cell infiltration into the tubulointerstitial area.

Arteriolar hyalinosis (Hyali): This is the percentage of hyalinc thickness of the whole arteriolar wall thickness. A totally occluded artery and an artery connecting to a globally sclerotic glomerulus are shown for comparison.

Intimal Thickening of Atherosclerosis (Athero) Fibrous intimal thickening of an arteriole or larger artery (interlobular artery, arcuate artery) together with the symmetrical wall should be evaluated. The branching artery is not assessed.

Figures 11.1 and 11.2 show the baseline pathological characteristics of the study group. GScle, IFTA, Hyali in red exhibited higher scores than those in G&Y and

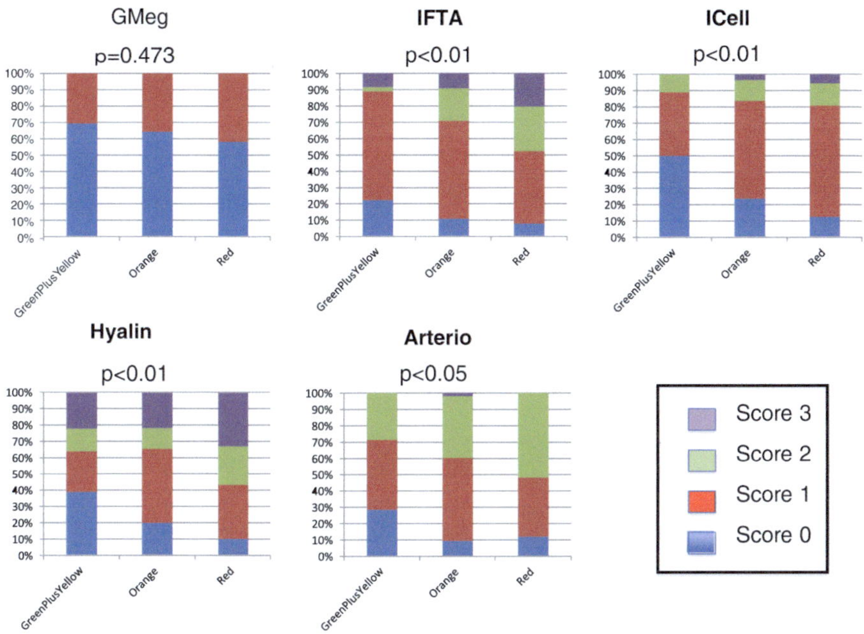

Fig. 11.1 The percent of each histological score in CKD heat map categories. GMeg: glomerulomegaly, IFTA: interstitial fibrosis and tubular atrophy, ICell: interstitial cell infiltration, Hyalin: arteriolar hyalinosis, Arterio: arteriosclerosis with intimal thickening. p was calculated by one-way ANOVA test [16]

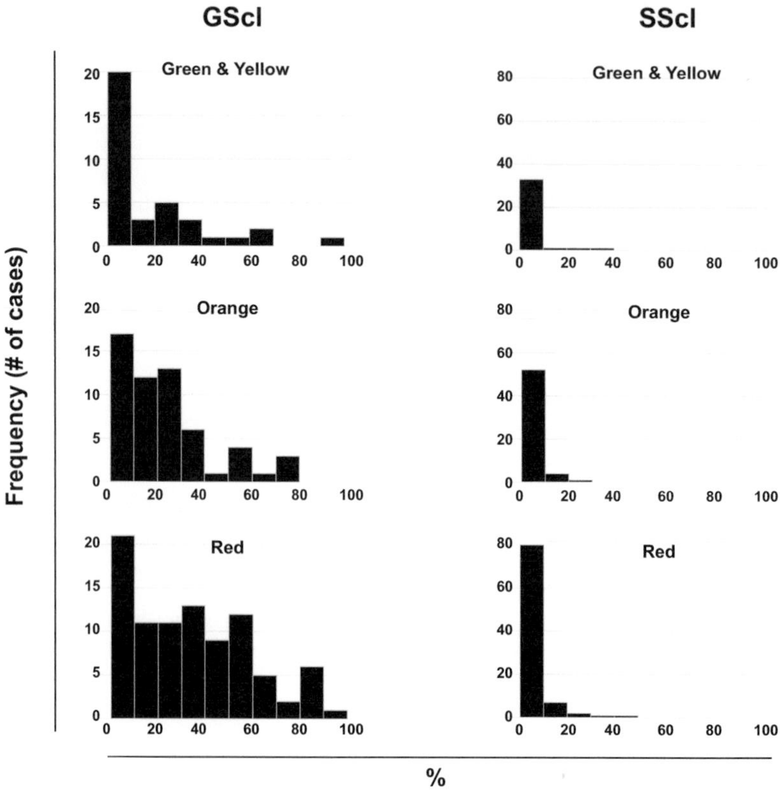

Fig. 11.2 Histogram of glomerular sclerosis in CKD heat map categories. GScl global glomerulosclerosis/collapsing glomerular change and ischemic glomerular change. *SScle* segmental glomerulosclerosis [16]

orange. Moreover, the scores of ICell and Athero in red and orange were also higher than those in G&Y. IFTA and Arterio lesions were observed in more than 70% of cases, even in the G&Y group. ICell and Hyali also progressed consistently with the progression of the heat map categories.

Then we checked the correlation between pathological findings and clinical findings (Table 11.2). GScle, IFTA, and Hyali were correlated with age. Aging leads to various anatomical and physiological changes of the kidney [18–20]. BMI, systolic BP, and diastolic BP were not correlated with pathologic factors.

Additionally, we looked at the association between clinicopathological features and several outcomes—commencement of dialysis, composite kidney events (commencement of dialysis, decrease of eGFR by ≥50%, or doubling of serum creatinine), cardiovascular events (cardiovascular death, nonfatal myocardial infarction, coronary interventions, or nonfatal stroke), and all-cause mortality. The incident rate of each outcome was reported with 95% confidence interval (CI).

Table 11.3 shows the incident rate of each outcome/100 person-years. The incidences of the composite kidney end points, dialysis, and all-cause mortality were

Table 11.2 Correlation between pathological findings and clinical findings

	GScle	SScle	GMega	IFTA	ICell	Hyali	Athero
Age	0.27*	0.14	0.14	0.19*	0.07	0.17*	0.12
BMI	−0.06	−0.03	0.07	0.01	0.00	0.00	−0.08
SysBP	0.04	0.10	0.10	0.05	0.06	0.08	0.07
DiaBP	0.02	−0.02	0.15	0.01	0.08	0.06	0.09
Cr	0.13	0.01	0.00	0.07	0.13	0.15	−0.04
Tcho	−0.13	−0.05	−0.08	−0.05	−0.06	−0.03	0.01
UAlb	−0.03	0.12	−0.03	−0.06	−0.03	−0.04	0.02
UOB	0.19*	−0.10	0.12	0.15*	0.06	0.09	−0.13

The number shown in the table is a correlation coefficient
BMI body mass index, *sysBP* systolic blood pressure, *diaBP* diastolic blood pressure, *Cr* creatinine, *Tcho* total cholesterol, *UAlb* urinary levels of albumin, *UOB* occult blood in urine
$^{*}p < 0.05$ [16]

Table 11.3 Incidence rates of each outcome/100 person-years

HeatMapGY	Green & Yellow			Orange			Red			Total		
	Rate	(95% Conf. Interval)		Rate	(95% Conf. Interval)		Rate	(95% Conf. Interval)		Rate	(95% Conf. Interval)	
Composite kidney event	1.42	0.53	3.79	2.16	1.03	4.54	3.98	2.69	5.89	2.92	2.11	4.05
Kidney death	0.00			0.00			0.61	0.20	1.90	0.31	0.10	0.95
CV event	1.64	0.41	6.56	0.97	0.14	6.91	1.49	0.56	3.96	1.42	0.68	2.97
All cause mortality	0.34	0.05	2.44	0.00			0.30	0.08	1.20	0.23	0.07	0.70

The composite kidney end point is defined as dialysis, doubling of Cr or halving of eGFR. Kidney death is defined as dialysis or kidney transplantation
CV event cardiovascular event [16]

significantly higher in higher-risk categories. Although the composite kidney end points (dialysis, doubling of Cr, or halving of eGFR) were observed in 36 patients, kidney death (dialysis or kidney transplantation), cardiovascular events, and death were only observed in three, seven, and three patients throughout the observation period, respectively.

Finally, the hazard ratio (HR) with 95% confidence interval (CI) for composite kidney end point was determined for various clinical and histological characteristics by Cox regression analysis.

Table 11.4 shows the results of the predictors in Cox analysis. In the univariate Cox analysis for the composite kidney end points, glomerular sclerosis, IFTA, and interstitial cell infiltration exhibited statistically significant high hazard ratios (1.18, 1.84, 1.69, respectively); placement in the red group of the CKD heat map categories also indicated a high hazard ratio (HR 2.85, $p = 0.053$). After adjustment for clinical and medication data, however, the association of glomerular sclerosis, IFTA, and interstitial cell infiltration with the composite kidney outcome did not remain significant in the multivariable Cox model. Only placement in the red group

Table 11.4 Cox analysis

	Univariate			Model 1			Model 2		
	HR	95% CI	*p*	HR	95% CI	*p*	HR	95% CI	*p*
Age	1.02	0.99–1.05	0.147	1.03	0.98–1.07	0.239	1.02	0.97–1.07	0.381
Gender	0.98	0.50–1.90	0.942	0.54	0.20–1.47	0.229	0.30	0.10–0.97	0.044
BMI	0.90	0.79–1.01	0.075	1.07	0.88–1.30	0.475	1.06	0.86–1.31	0.562
SysBP	1.01	0.99–1.02	0.450	1.03	1.00–1.05	0.068	1.02	0.99–1.05	0.130
Tcho	1.00	1.00–1.00	0.720	1.00	1.00–1.00	0.896	1.00	1.00–1.00	0.754
UOB	1.35	0.90–2.04	0.152	1.26	0.67–2.37	0.466	1.41	0.75–2.66	0.286
eGFR	0.97	0.95–0.99	0.005						
Ualb	1.03	0.95–1.12	0.483						
HeatMapGY									
G&Y	Ref			Ref			Ref		
Orange	1.37	0.40–4.74	0.619	5.48	0.51–58.88	0.160	4.77	0.43–52.78	0.203
Red	2.85	0.99–8.24	0.053	9.58	1.08–84.55	0.042	9.51	1.03–87.96	0.047
RASI	1.72	0.76–3.91	0.195				1.22	0.27–5.46	0.793
LipidDrug	1.93	0.97–3.84	0.061				0.23	0.03–1.76	0.157
CCB	1.58	0.53–4.72	0.413				3.60	0.95–13.67	0.060
GScle/10%	1.18	1.04–1.33	0.010	1.04	0.83–1.30	0.730	0.98	0.78–1.23	0.847
SScle/10%	1.28	0.84–1.95	0.249						
GMega	1.63	0.76–3.48	0.210						
IFTA	1.84	1.22–2.77	0.004	1.92	0.74–4.99	0.178	2.03	0.76–5.40	0.155
ICell	1.69	1.12–2.56	0.013	0.83	0.32–2.15	0.705	0.88	0.32–2.37	0.794
Hyali	1.30	0.91–1.85	0.145						
Athero	1.39	0.82–2.36	0.222						

Model 1; Adjusted by age, gender, body mass index, systolic blood pressure, serum levels of total cholesterol, urinary occult blood, NSGScle, NSIFTA, NSICell, and HeatMapG&Y. Model 2; adjusted by Model 1 + RAS3, LipidDrug, and CCB [16]

was a statistically significant risk factor for the composite kidney end points (HR 9.51).

In summary, although some pathological findings, such as IFTA and atherosclerosis, were observed even in cases with preserved eGFR and a small amount of albuminuria (G&Y categories), pathological findings had minor impacts on prediction of the composite kidney outcomes in this study.

11.2 Nephrosclerosis and Diabetic Nephropathy

It is well known that the hallmarks of typical diabetic nephropathy are basement thickening and nodular lesion in mesangial matrix (Kimmelstiel-Wilson lesion) [21, 22]. Both are featured by the accumulation of extracellular matrix, which has been considered as a consequence of long-standing diabetes. These lesions cannot be usually seen in nephrosclerosis. On the other hand, it is considered that nephrosclerosis and diabetic nephropathy share various pathological features, since both are chronic lifestyle-related diseases that affect elderly people as well as those with hyperglycemia, hypertension, obesity, and/or dyslipidemia. However, this has not been confirmed. Indeed, the biopsy-based studies comparing nephrosclerosis and diabetic nephropathy are lacking.

Against this background, the present study was performed to examine similarities and differences in pathological lesions between nephrosclerosis and diabetic nephropathy.

We present the data in which obtained from the two retrospective studies done with 184 patients with biopsy-proven nephrosclerosis and 600 patients with biopsy-proven diabetic nephropathy, in 13 centers across Japan [17, 23].

Table 11.5 shows the pathological findings of nephrosclerosis and diabetic nephropathy. We found that nephrosclerosis and diabetic nephropathy share pathological features in interstitial and vascular lesions but not in all glomerular lesions. In glomerular lesions, several lesions such as diffuse lesion (mesangial lesion), nodular lesion (nodular sclerosis), subendothelial space widening (double contour of exudative lesion), mesangiolysis/microaneurysm, and peri-hilar neovascularization (polar vasculosis) can be seen only in diabetic nephropathy.

Table 11.6 shows the pathological score of nephrosclerosis and diabetic nephropathy. The severity of IFTA, interstitial inflammation, and arteriolar sclerosis was higher in diabetic nephropathy compared to nephrosclerosis as the CKD heat map categorization goes up.

Table 11.5 Pathological findings of diabetic nephropathy and nephrosclerosis

Pathological findings of *diabetic nephropathy and nephrosclerosis*

	Pathologic findings
Glomerular lesions	Diffuse lesion (mesangial expansion)
	Nodular lesion (nodular sclerosis)
	Subendothelial space widening (double contour of basement membrane)
	Exudative lesion
	Mesangiolysis/microaneurysm
	Peri-hilar neo-vascularization (polar vasculosis)
	Global glomerulosclerosis/collapsing glomerulopathy·ischemic nephropathy
	Segmental glomerulosclerosis
	Glomerulomegaly
Interstitial lesions	Interstitial fibrosis and tubular atrophy (IFTA)
	Interstitial inflammation
Vascular lesions	Arteriolar hyalinosis
	Intimal thickening

Pathological findings of *diabetic nephropathy* (Diffuse lesion through Intimal thickening)

Pathological findings of *nephrosclerosis* (Global glomerulosclerosis through Intimal thickening)

Furuichi et al. [16, 23]

Table 11.6 Pathological scores of diabetic nephropathy and nephrosclerosis

CKD by GFR and albuminuria category	G&Y		Orange		Red		(Mean) Total	
	Nephrosclerosis	Diabetic nephropathy	Nephrosclerosis	Diabetic nephropathy	Nephrosclerosis	Diabetic nephropathy	Nephrosclerosis	Diabetic nephropathy
Global glomerulosclerosis	17.62	8.21*	22.78	17.09	33.28	32.44	26.96	24.36
Segmental glomerulosclerosis	2.19	2.16	1.87	2.66	3.28	4.74	2.63	3.77
Glomerulomegaly	0.31	0.22	0.36	0.31	0.42	0.40	0.38	0.35
Interstitial fibrosis and tubular atrophy	0.97	0.88	1.27	1.42	1.60	2.17*	1.37	1.76*
Interstitial inflammation	0.61	0.75	0.96	1.05	1.12	1.53*	0.97	1.27*
Arteriolar hyalinosis	1.19	1.50	1.36	2.05*	1.80	2.36*	1.54	2.13*
Intimal thickening	1.00	0.87	1.32	1.09	1.40	1.38	1.29	1.22

Furuichi et al. [16, 23]
T test
Data from Ref. [16] and [19]
*$p < 0.05$ to nephrosclerosis

In summary, although nephrosclerosis and diabetic nephropathy share various pathological features, several glomerular lesions such as diffuse lesion (mesangial lesion), nodular lesion (nodular sclerosis), subendothelial space widening (double contour of exudative lesion), mesangiolysis/microaneurysm, and peri-hilar neovascularization (polar vasculosis) can be seen only in diabetic nephropathy.

References

1. Jha V, Garcia-Garcia G, Iseki K, Li Z, Naicker S, Plattner B, Saran R, Wang AY, Yang CW. Chronic kidney disease: global dimension and perspectives. Lancet. 2013;382(9888):260–72. https://doi.org/10.1016/S0140-6736(13)60687-X. Erratum in: Lancet. 2013;382(9888):208.
2. United States Renal Data System. 2016 USRDS annual data report: epidemiology of kidney disease in the United States. Bethesda, MD: National Institutes of Health, National Institute of Diabetes and Digestive and Kidney Diseases; 2016.
3. ERA-EDTA Registry. ERA-EDTA Registry annual report 2015. Amsterdam: Academic Medical Center, Department of Medical Informatics; 2017.
4. Japanese Society for Dialysis Therapy Renal Data Registry. Annual report 2014, JSDT Renal Data Registry (JRDR). Ren Replace Ther 2014;3:18. https://doi.org/10.1186/s41100-017-0097-8.
5. Takebayashi S, Kiyoshi Y, Hisano S, Uesugi N, Sasatomi Y, Meng J, Sakata N. Benign nephrosclerosis: incidence, morphology and prognosis. Clin Nephrol. 2001;55(5):349–56.
6. Liang S, Le W, Liang D, Chen H, Xu F, Chen H, Liu Z, Zeng C. Clinico-pathological characteristics and outcomes of patients with biopsy-proven hypertensive nephrosclerosis: a retrospective cohort study. BMC Nephrol. 2016;17:42. https://doi.org/10.1186/s12882-016-0254-2.
7. Haruhara K, Tsuboi N, Kanzaki G, Koike K, Suyama M, Shimizu A, Miyazaki Y, Kawamura T, Ogura M, Yokoo T. Glomerular density in biopsy-proven hypertensive nephrosclerosis. Am J Hypertens. 2015;28(9):1164–71. https://doi.org/10.1093/ajh/hpu267.
8. Olson JL. Renal disease caused by hypertension. In: Jenette JC, Olson JL, Schwartz MM, Silva FG, editors. Heptinstall's pathology of the kidney. 7th ed. Philadelphia: Wolters Kluwer; 2015. p. 849–96.
9. Morduchowicz G, Boner G, Ben-Bassat M, Rosenfeld JB. Proteinuria in benign nephrosclerosis. Arch Intern Med. 1986;146(8):1513–6.
10. Narvarte J, Privé M, Saba SR, Ramirez G. Proteinuria in hypertension. Am J Kidney Dis. 1987;10(6):408–16.
11. Toto RD. Proteinuria and hypertensive nephrosclerosis in African Americans. Kidney Int Suppl. 2004;92:S102–4.
12. Dasgupta I, Porter C, Innes A, Burden R. "Benign" hypertensive nephrosclerosis. QJM. 2007;100(2):113–9.
13. Vikse BE, Aasarød K, Bostad L, Iversen BM. Clinical prognostic factors in biopsy-proven benign nephrosclerosis. Nephrol Dial Transplant. 2003;18(3):517–23.
14. Sumida K, Hoshino J, Ueno T, Mise K, Hayami N, Suwabe T, Kawada M, Imafuku A, Hiramatsu R, Hasegawa E, Yamanouchi M, Sawa N, Fujii T, Ohashi K, Takaichi K, Ubara Y. Effect of proteinuria and glomerular filtration rate on renal outcome in patients with biopsy-proven benign nephrosclerosis. PLoS One. 2016;11(1):e0147690. https://doi.org/10.1371/journal.pone.0147690.
15. Momoki K, Kataoka H, Moriyama T, Mochizuki T, Nitta K. Hyperuricemia as a predictive marker for progression of nephrosclerosis: clinical assessment of prognostic factors in biopsy-proven arterial/arteriolar nephrosclerosis. J Atheroscler Thromb. 2017;24(6):630–42. https://doi.org/10.5551/jat.37523.

16. Furuichi K, Shimizu M, Yuzawa Y, Hara A, Toyama T, Kitamura H, Suzuki Y, Sato H, Uesugi N, Ubara Y, Hoshino J, Hisano S, Ueda Y, Nishi S, Yokoyama H, Nishino T, Kohagura K, Ogawa D, Mise K, Shibagaki Y, Kimura K, Haneda M, Makino H, Matsuo S, Wada T, Research Group of Diabetic Nephropathy and Nephrosclerosis, Ministry of Health, Labour and Welfare of Japan, and Japan Agency for Medical Research and Development. Nationwide multicenter kidney biopsy study of Japanese patients with hypertensive nephrosclerosis. Clin Exp Nephrol. 2017;22(3):629–37. https://doi.org/10.1007/s10157-017-1496-4.
17. Levin A, Stevens PE. Summary of KDIGO 2012 CKD Guideline: behind the scenes, need for guidance, and a framework for moving forward. Kidney Int. 2014;85(1):49–61. https://doi.org/10.1038/ki.2013.444.
18. Glassock RJ, Rule AD. The implications of anatomical and functional changes of the aging kidney: with an emphasis on the glomeruli. Kidney Int. 2012;82(3):270–7. https://doi.org/10.1038/ki.2012.65.
19. O'Sullivan ED, Hughes J, Ferenbach DA. Renal aging: causes and consequences. J Am Soc Nephrol. 2017;28(2):407–20. https://doi.org/10.1681/ASN.2015121308.
20. Hommos MS, Glassock RJ, Rule AD. Structural and functional changes in human kidneys with healthy aging. J Am Soc Nephrol. 2017;28(10):2838–44. https://doi.org/10.1681/ASN.2017040421.
21. Olson JL, Laszik ZG. Diabetic nephropathy. In: Jenette JC, Olson JL, Schwartz MM, Silva FG, editors. Heptinstall's pathology of the kidney. 7th ed. Philadelphia: Wolters Kluwer; 2015. p. 897–949.
22. Tervaert TW, Mooyaart AL, Amann K, Cohen AH, Cook HT, Drachenberg CB, Ferrario F, Fogo AB, Haas M, de Heer E, Joh K, Noël LH, Radhakrishnan J, Seshan SV, Bajema IM, Bruijn JA. Renal pathology society. Pathologic classification of diabetic nephropathy. J Am Soc Nephrol. 2010;21(4):556–63. https://doi.org/10.1681/ASN.2010010010.
23. Furuichi K, Yuzawa Y, Shimizu M, Hara A, Toyama T, Kitamura H, Suzuki Y, Sato H, Uesugi N, Ubara Y, Hisano S, Ueda Y, Nishi S, Yokoyama H, Nishino T, Kohagura K, Ogawa D, Mise K, Shibagaki Y, Kimura K, Haneda M, Makino H, Matsuo S, Wada T. Nationwide multicentre kidney biopsy study of Japanese patients with type 2 diabetes. Nephrol Dial Transplant. 2017;33(1) https://doi.org/10.1093/ndt/gfw417.

Chapter 12
Nondiabetic Renal Disease (NDRD) and Diabetic Kidney Disease (DKD)

Koki Mise

Background

More Heterogeneous DKD Leads to Difficulty in Differentiating DN Alone from NDRD Superimposed on DN

Diabetes mellitus (DM) remains the primary cause of end-stage renal disease (ESRD) requiring renal replacement therapy in many parts of the world, and the coexistence of DM and kidney disease amplifies the risk of mortality and cardiovascular disease [1, 2]. Among the US adults, the prevalence of chronic kidney disease (CKD) in patients with type 2 diabetes mellitus (T2DM) was reported to be three times higher than in the nondiabetic population [3]. Unlike clinical course of diabetic kidney disease (DKD) in patients with type 1 diabetes mellitus (T1DM), that in patients with T2DM appears to be more complicated and heterogeneous [4, 5]. This is because patients with T2DM tend to have more metabolic complications compared to those with T1DM, and the clinical manifestations of patients with T2DM vary in different countries and races [6, 7], as well as the treatments for T2DM can influence clinical course of DKD [8–11].

Scheme of relationships among CKD with diabetes, DKD, and diabetic nephropathy (DN; which was defined as diabetes-induced renal disease confirmed histologically) in patients with diabetes and/or CKD is shown in Fig. 12.1a, b. Actual size of each disease category remains unclear because of the recent heterogeneous manifestations of DKD and DN. The group of CKD with diabetes includes not only DKD/DN but also nondiabetic renal disease (NDRD), and DKD often coexists with nephrosclerosis (Fig. 12.1a) [12]. Basically, Fig. 12.1a shows the true relationship among groups since the definition of CKD includes structural change or abnormality, suggesting histologically confirmed renal disease [13].

K. Mise (✉)
Department of Nephrology, Rheumatology, Endocrinology and Metabolism, Okayama University Graduate School of Medicine, Dentistry and Pharmaceutical Sciences, Okayama, Japan
e-mail: kokims-frz@okayama-u.ac.jp

T. Wada et al. (eds.), *Diabetic Kidney Disease*,
https://doi.org/10.1007/978-981-15-9301-7_12

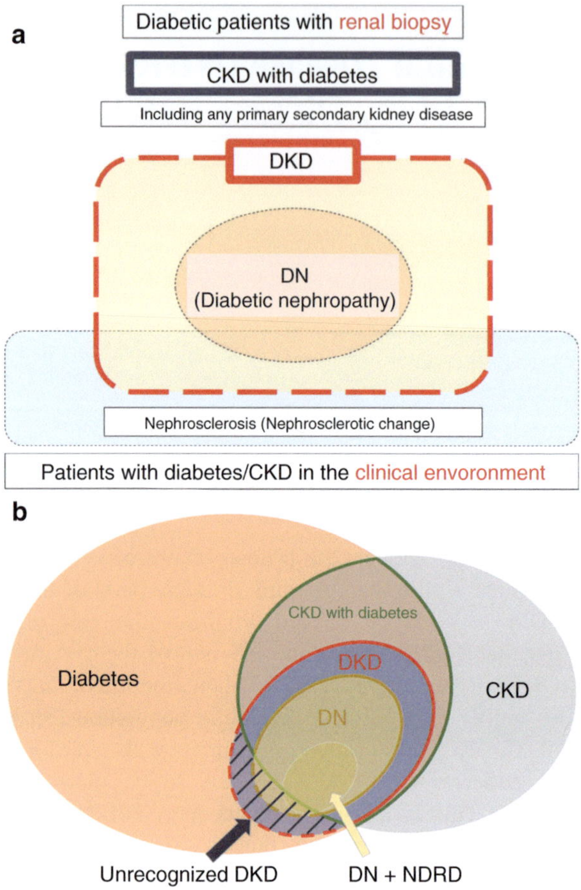

Fig. 12.1 (**a**) Scheme of the relationships CKD with diabetes, DKD, and DN in patients who underwent renal biopsy, modified from Furuichi et al. [12]. (**b**) Scheme of the relationships among diabetes, CKD, DKD, and DN in the clinical environment. The definition of "DKD" is still controversial, but it seems that most nephrologists regard DKD as chronic kidney diseases whose etiology is diabetes and its related factors. DN classically implicates histologically confirmed renal disease induced by diabetes. In clinical practice, there is a selection bias in diabetic patients who undergo renal biopsy, and the indication of renal biopsy in patients with diabetes varies among institutions. In addition, clinical manifestations of DKD are becoming more heterogeneous than before. Recently, nephrosclerosis (nephrosclerotic changes) on renal tissue of DKD is often observed. Thus, the true scheme size of each category remains unknown and might be variable in countries and races. Abbreviations: *CKD* chronic kidney disease, *DKD* diabetic kidney disease, *DN* diabetic nephropathy

However, in the clinical environment, a part of DKD is unrecognized because it has not been confirmed by renal biopsy and is not classified into CKD (Fig. 12.1b). Clinically, most renal biopsy in patients with DM is performed to differentiate from NDRD [14, 15]. We usually consider the renal biopsy in patients with DM and atypical clinical course or manifestation, and the "atypical" or "typical" is left to the judgment of each physician. Because of the unstandardized indication of renal biopsy in patients with DM, little is unknown about what NDRDs are likely superimposed on DN and what kind of clinical manifestations are actually useful to differentiate NDRDs and to consider subsequent renal biopsy. Research renal biopsy in patients with DM is needed to answer these clinical questions, whereas evidences for the clinical questions are limited to the studies based on clinical biopsy in each institution, except for few studies of research biopsy with small number of diabetic patients.

In this section, (1) NDRD superimposed on DN and (2) predictors for differentiating among DN alone, coexistence of NDRD, and NDRD alone are summarized in terms of the clinicopathologic results from recent studies in which clinical biopsy was performed in patients with DM, especially T2DM.

12.1 NDRD Superimposed on DN

12.1.1 Prevalence and the Most Common NDRD

Recently, ERA-EDTA Immunonephrology Working Group performed systematic review and meta-analysis of 48 studies (4876 diabetic patients) for clarifying the potential usefulness of renal biopsy in patients with diabetes [2]. The characteristic of this meta-analysis was that the most studies were retrospective in design (75%), were performed in Asian countries (27/48 studies, 46% of total patients), and had patients with T2DM (83%). More importantly, only 3% of diabetic patients included in this analysis underwent research renal biopsy. In the present study, the prevalence of DN, NDRD, and mixed forms (DN + NDRD) was extremely variable, ranging from 6.5 to 94%, 3 to 82.9%, and 4 to 45.5% of the overall diagnosis, respectively.

Immunoglobulin A (IgA) nephropathy was the most frequent NDRD in 16 studies, followed by membranous nephropathy (MN) in nine studies [2], and the two renal diseases were the majority of NDRD in other studies and a review published after the meta-analysis [16–18]. However, high prevalence of Asian populations in the meta-analysis could influence these results as discussed in the article [2]. Intriguingly, among 2619 patients enrolled in 19 studies except for studies from Asian countries, focal-segmental glomerulosclerosis (FSGS) was the most frequent NDRD (11%), followed by IgA nephropathy (9%), and MN (8%). Especially, FSGS was predominant in the studies from the USA. Similarly, in another study from New Zealand, FSGS was the most common NDRD in patients with T2DM (78 patients (46%) out of 169 patients with NDRD or mixed forms), and the 66% of participants included in the study were Maori and Pasifika patients [19].

Therefore, the most common NDRD in patients with diabetes (especially T2DM) who clinically need renal biopsy might be IgA nephropathy in Asian countries and FSGS in other countries, although it could vary in areas and races.

12.1.2 Renal Prognosis and Mortality Among DN, NDRD, and Mixed Forms

There have been few studies in which renal prognosis of DN alone, NDRD superimposed on DN (mixed forms), and NDRD alone was directly compared. Oh et al. reported that the renal prognosis was the worst in the group of patients with DN alone among the three groups (Fig. 12.2a) [20]. The estimated renal survival rate at 5 years after renal biopsy was 61.7% in patients with DN alone, 81.8% in those with mixed forms, and 89.2% in those with NDRD. In this study, IgA

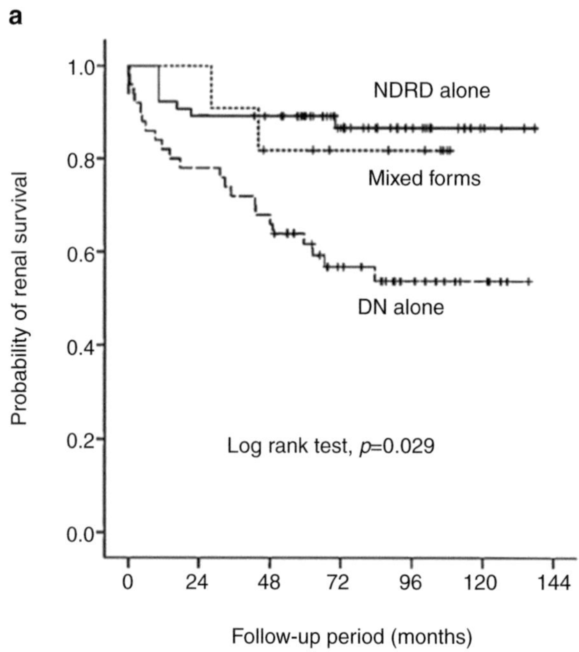

Fig. 12.2 (**a–c**) Renal survival rate among patients with DN alone, mixed forms, and NDRD alone. (**a**) Modified from Oh et al. [20]. (**b**) Modified from Chang et al. [21]. (**c**) Modified from Tan et al. [19]. (**d**) Modified from Wang et al. [17]. Endpoint was end-stage renal disease in all analyses. In the analysis of (**c**), renal survival estimates were adjusted for age, ethnicity, body mass index, gender, proteinuria, and estimated glomerular filtration rate at the time of renal biopsy. Overall, patients with DN alone had worse renal prognosis compared with those with NDRD alone. On the other hand, the renal prognosis in patients with mixed forms varies among studies, which might result from the different severity of DN superimposed on NDRD and different clinical parameters at baseline. (**e**) Cumulative overall survival rates among patients with DN alone, mixed forms, and NDRD alone. Modified from Tan et al. [19]. In this analysis, overall survival rates were adjusted for age, ethnicity, body mass index, gender, proteinuria, and estimated glomerular filtration rate at the time of renal biopsy. During the median follow-up of 3.6 years, the overall survival was significantly poorer in patients with DN alone than in patients with NDRD (NDRD alone and mixed forms) ($P = 0.025$)

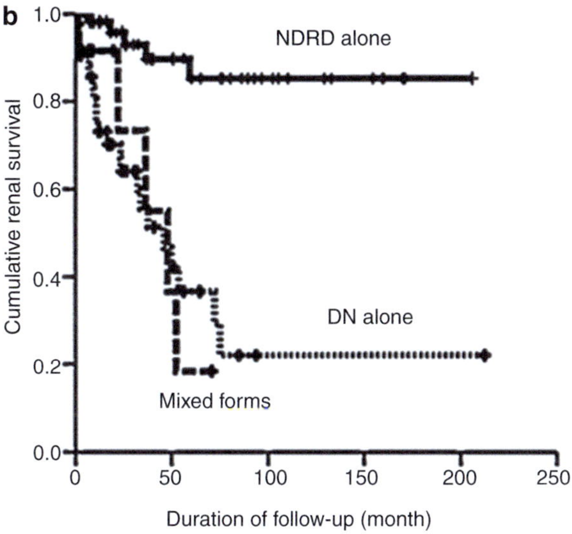

NDRD vs DN (DN alone + mixed forms): $P<0.001$
Mixed forms vs DN alone: $P>0.05$

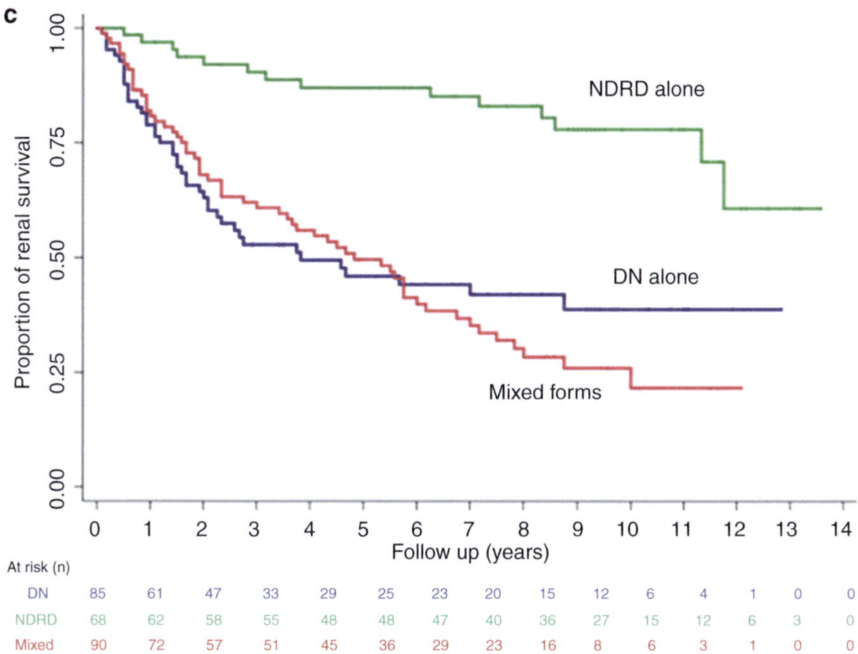

NDRD vs DN (DN alone + mixed forms): $P<0.001$
Mixed forms vs DN alone: $P>0.05$

Fig. 12.2 (continued)

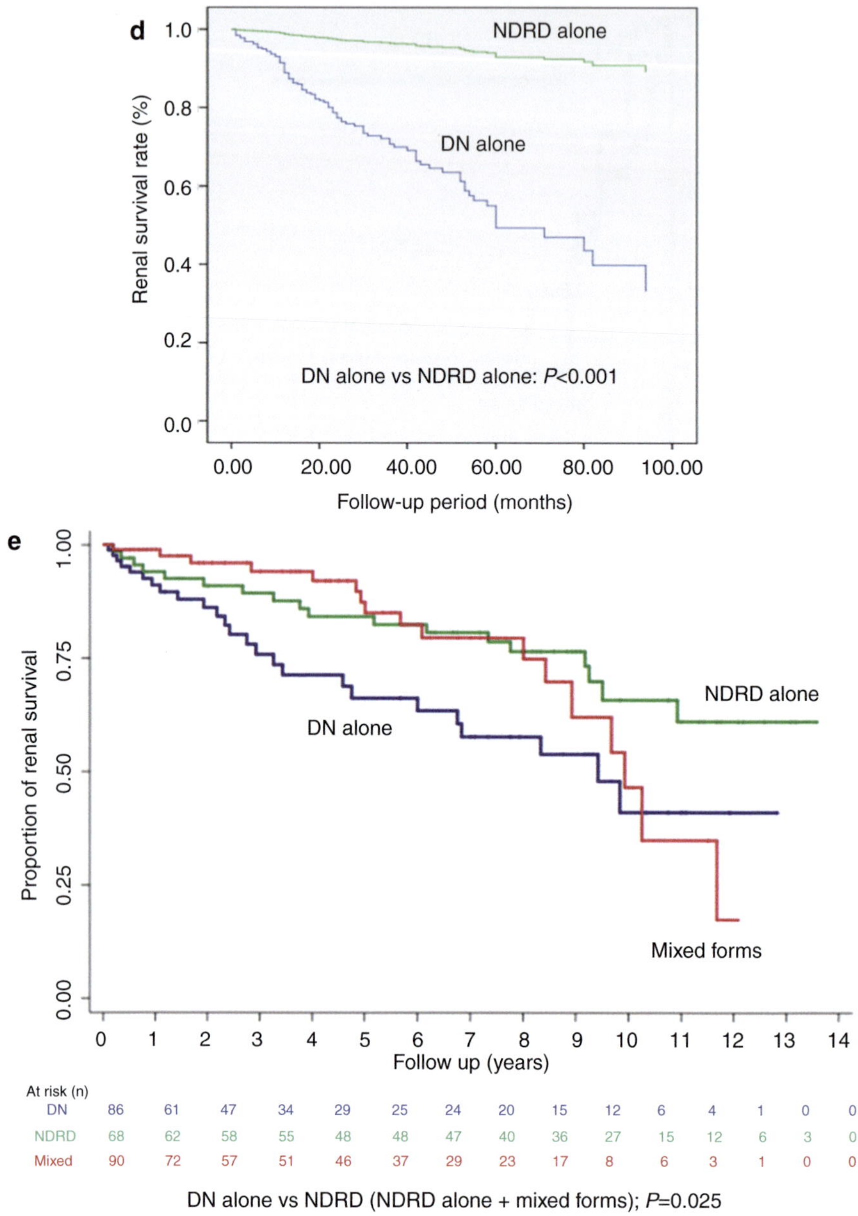

Fig. 12.2 (continued)

nephropathy was the most frequent coexisting NDRD, and it was present in nine patients with NDRD alone and in seven patients with mixed forms. The second common NDRD was MN, and it was found in 13 patients with NDRD alone and in two patients with mixed forms.

Meanwhile, another Korean study revealed that there was not significant difference of renal prognosis between DN alone and mixed forms (Fig. 12.2b) [21]. MN was the most frequent kidney disease except for DN in the study, and it was observed in 19 patients with NDRD alone and in six patients with mixed forms. Minimal change disease which was the second dominant NDRD was observed in 12 patients with sole NDRD. IgA nephropathy was found in eight patients with NDRD alone and in one patient with mixed forms.

Similar results were observed in the other cohort study from New Zealand (Fig. 12.2c) [19]. The median rate of eGFR slope in the NDRD group was significantly slower at 2.2 (interquartile range [IQR] −0.1–5.8) mL/min/1.73 m^2/year than the DN alone group and mixed form group (8.3 [IQR 3.0–17.2] and 6.9 [IQR 2.0–12.4] mL/min/1.73 m^2/year, respectively, $P < 0.001$). In addition to the results of renal prognosis, all-cause mortality was compared among these three groups [19]. As well as the renal prognosis, the overall survival was poorest in patients with DN alone during median 3.6 years of follow-up (log-rank test, $P = 0.025$, Fig. 12.2e). The characteristic finding of this study was that the most common NDRD was FSGS (46% in patients with NDRD or mixed forms) and the second one was interstitial nephritis (24%).

In the more recent study with large number of T2DM patients, the renal prognosis was compared between the group of 302 patients with DN alone and the group of 174 patients with NDRD alone [17]. The renal prognosis defined as ESRD was significantly worse in patients with DN alone ($P < 0.001$, Fig. 12.2d). Importantly, in all of the abovementioned studies, baseline renal function such as eGFR and creatinine clearance rate was already lower in DN alone group compared with NDRD group [17, 19–21]. Nevertheless, intriguingly, DN alone was significantly associated with ESRD independent of baseline eGFR and proteinuria in the latest study (Hazard ratio for DN alone 6.687, 95% confidence interval 3.137–14.258, $P = 0.001$) [17].

Given these results, it seems that the renal prognosis of DN is commonly worse compared with that of NDRD alone, whereas the renal prognosis of mixed forms is variable. This might result from the different severities of DN superimposed on NDRD rather than the different kinds of NDRD superimposed on DN although the details of histopathological severity of DN in patients with NDRD and mixed forms were not shown in the abovementioned studies [19–21]. In addition, the best renal prognosis in patients with NDRD alone might reflect that detection of NDRD by renal biopsy leads to the subsequent successful treatment to each NDRD.

12.2 Predictors for Differentiating Among DN Alone, Coexistence of NDRD, and NDRD Alone

12.2.1 Duration of DM

Clinical determinants for differentiating among DN alone, coexistence of NDRD, and NDRD alone have been investigated in many studies. A retrospective cross-sectional study from Columbia University Medical Center showed that 23.5% (620 patients) of 2642 patients who underwent renal biopsy were diabetics [22]. In addition, among 611 diabetic patients with adequate tissue for diagnosis, 227 patients (37%) were diagnosed with DN alone, 164 (27%) were diagnosed with DN plus NDRD (mixed forms), and 220 (36%) were diagnosed with NDRD alone.

Multivariate logistic regression analysis to assess the useful predictors of NDRD (including mixed forms and NDRD alone) versus DN alone revealed that longer duration of DM was only significantly associated with a greater likelihood of DN alone and lower likelihood of all NDRD (odds ratio [OR] for NDRD, 0.95; 95% confidence interval [CI], 0.91–0.98; $P = 0.004$, Table 12.1). DM duration ≥12 years was the best predictor of DN alone (sensitivity 57.5%, specificity 73.3%, positive predictive value 56.0%, negative predictive value 74.5%, and AUC 0.66 [95% CI 0.60–0.73]), and DM duration ≥8 years was the best predictor of all DN including NDRD superimposed on DN (sensitivity 76.8%, specificity 63.2%, positive predictive value 78.5%, negative predictive value 61.0%, and AUC 0.75 [95% CI 0.69–0.81]). In secondary analyses, nephrotic-range proteinuria was also inversely associated with finding NDRD alone (OR for NDRD alone, 0.32 [95% CI 0.11–0.95; $P = 0.04$]).

These results might suggest that renal biopsy should be considered for identifying NDRD if a diabetic patient whose duration of DM no more than 12 years has urine abnormalities. Similarly, usefulness of short duration of DM for predicting NDRD was reported in many studies [17, 18, 21, 23–25]. However, whether sensitivity and specificity of short DM duration is enough to predict NDRD remains controversial.

12.2.2 Diabetic Retinopathy

Diabetic retinopathy is one of three major complications of DM, and the development of diabetic retinopathy is related with long and poor glycemic control, as well as DN [26, 27]. Many previous studies demonstrated that presence of diabetic retinopathy was an independent predictor of the renal prognosis of DN [7, 28, 29], suggesting that it could be a predictor of existence of DN.

In the abovementioned study from Columbia University, degree of proteinuria, baseline eGFR, age, gender, race, duration of DM, acute kidney injury, serum complement levels, and serum and urine protein electrophoresis were selected as potential confounders in the multivariate logistic regression analysis, whereas

Table 12.1 Association of key clinical predictors and biopsy findings of NDRD

Variables	OR (95% CI)	*P* Value
Proteinuria (mg/d)		
<500	1.00 (reference)	
500–3500	1.28 (0.39–4.20)	0.68
>3500	0.55 (0.19–1.66)	0.29
eGFR (mL/min/1.73 m^2)		
>60	1.00 (reference)	
30–60	0.89 (0.35–2.25)	0.81
15–30	1.42(0.53–3.82)	0.49
≤15	1.54 (0.48–4.96)	0.47
Age	1.03 (1.00–1.06)	0.06
Male sex	1.05 (0.54–2.02)	0.89
Race		
Unknown	1.00 (reference)	
White	0.93 (0.46–1.91)	0.85
Black	1.38 (0.49–3.84)	0.54
Hispanic	1.07 (0.27–4.23)	0.93
Asian	1.66 (0.26–10.67)	0.59
Duration of diabetes	0.95 (0.91–0.98)	0.004
AKI	1.44 (0.67–3.07)	0.35
Low complements	4.70 (0.49–45.42)	0.18
M-spike (serum or urine)	1.50 (0.51–4.37)	0.46

Modified from Sharma et al. [22]

In this multivariate logistic regression analysis to assess the useful predictors of NDRD (including NDRD plus DN) versus DN alone, longer duration of DM was only significantly associated with a greater likelihood of DN alone and lower likelihood of all NDRD (OR for NDRD, 0.95 [95% CI 0.91–0.98], $P = 0.004$)

Abbreviation: *OR* odds ratio, *CI* confidence interval, *eGFR* estimated glomerular filtration rate, *AKI* acute kidney injury

diabetic retinopathy was not included in it [22]. Diabetic retinopathy was also reported to be a useful predictor for differentiating DN alone from NDRD in many previous studies [17, 21, 23–25, 30].

Among 97 Japanese patients with T2DM manifesting over proteinuria who underwent renal biopsy, 35 patients (36%) had DN alone, 16 patients (17%) had NDRD superimposed on DN, and 46 (47%) had NDRD alone [23]. Four clinical parameters such as duration of DM, diabetic retinopathy, microscopic hematuria, and granular casts in urinary sediment were used for analysis to check the clinically utility to differentiate NDRD from DN alone. Absence of any type of diabetic retinopathy showed the highest sensitivity (93%) and specificity (87%) among four parameters, although short duration of DM also showed high sensitivity (70%) and specificity (75%) (Table 12.2).

Similar results were confirmed in two studies from Asian countries. Chang et al. reported that multivariate logistic regression analysis revealed that absence of

Table 12.2 The sensitivity and specificity for discriminating NDRD (including mixed forms and NDRD alone) from DN alone

Clinical parameters	Sensitivity (%)	Specificity (%)	Likelihood ratio
Short duration of diabetes (<5 years) [vs. duration of diabetes ≥5 years]	70	75	2.81
Absence of diabetic retinopathy [vs. presence of diabetic retinopathy]	93	87	7.14
Presence of microscopic hematuria [vs. absence of microscopic hematuria]	69	56	1.57
Presence of granular cast [vs. absence of granular cast]	47	68	1.46

Modified from Tone et al. [23]

Among patients with any type of diabetic retinopathy, 83.3% (20/24) belonged to the DN alone group, and among patients without diabetic retinopathy, 94.7% (54/57) had NDRD. On the other hand, among the patients who had short duration of diabetes (defined as <5 years), 84.6 % (33/39) of the patients had NDRD. There were 26 patients with NDRD (77%) among 47 patients with microscopic hematuria

diabetic retinopathy was an independent predictor of NDRD in patients with T2DM and clinical manifestations of renal disease (OR 10.83 [95% CI 2.67–43.9], $P < 0.01$) after adjusting for age, the presence of hypertension, serum creatinine levels, hemoglobin levels, and duration of DM [21]. Likely, the study including 476 T2DM patients with DN alone or NDRD alone from China revealed that presence of diabetic retinopathy was an independent predictor of DN alone in the multivariate model (OR 4.171 [95% CI 1.810–9.612], $P = 0.001$) [17].

Based on these results, renal biopsy might be recommended for detecting NDRD in diabetic patients with clinical manifestations of renal disease but diabetic retinopathy.

12.2.3 Hematuria

In general, hematuria is not observed in typical and early DN, and the presence of hematuria is associated with more advanced DN although it was not significantly associated with renal prognosis independently of established clinical factors [7]. In Asian countries, IgA nephropathy is the most frequent NDRD, and the most common presenting finding of IgA nephropathy is hematuria. Accordingly, hematuria can be a useful determinant for differentiating DN alone and NDRD, especially in Asian countries.

Recent meta-analysis including 35 articles with 4005 diabetic patients demonstrated that diagnostic OR, the pooled sensitivity, and the specificity for the presence of hematuria to detect NDRD were 1.85 (95% CI 1.49–2.30), 0.42 (95%CI 0.35–0.49), and 0.72 (0.64–0.79), respectively [31]. In addition, area under the summary receiver operating characteristic curve (SROC-AUC) was 0.59 (0.54–0.63), while the positive likelihood ratio and negative likelihood ratio were 1.49 (1.28–1.75) and 0.81 (0.75–0.87), respectively.

On the other hand, another meta-analysis for five articles included in the same study revealed that the presence of dysmorphic red blood cell showed high specificity for predicting NDRD (0.94, 95%CI 0.91–0.97), and SROC-AUC was 0.79 (95%CI 0.75–0.82), although the pooled sensitivity was 0.27 (95%CI 0.23–0.32) [31].

Based on these results, hematuria has a certain level of predictive ability for differentiating NDRD from DN alone. In clinical practice, adding hematuria to other useful clinical predictors including diabetic retinopathy and duration of DM might improve predictive power. Indeed, Zhou et al. demonstrated that a model containing diabetes duration, diabetic retinopathy, hematuria, systolic blood pressure, and HbA1c clearly discriminated DN from NDRD (sensitivity 90%, specificity 92%, positive predictive value 93%, negative predictive value 89%, and total consistency 91%) [32].

In summary, short duration of DM, absence of diabetic retinopathy, and presence of hematuria can be useful predictors for differentiating NDRD from DN alone. Moreover, combination of these factors might further improve the ability of discrimination. However, all of the results shown in this section derived from clinical biopsy studies, and the indication of renal biopsy was variable, which may suggest that most cases of DN alone in these studies were regarded as "atypical" and "need for renal biopsy" by each primary doctor or department. Therefore, it might be difficult to apply these results to the clinical practice in all diabetic patients with CKD. The problem of selection bias is perennial in the studies based on clinical renal biopsy [33, 34], so further investigation of research biopsy with large number of diabetic patients is warranted.

References

1. Caramori ML. Should all patients with diabetes have a kidney biopsy? Nephrol Dial Transplant. 2017;32:3–5.
2. Fiorentino M, Bolignano D, Tesar V, Pisano A, Biesen WV, Tripepi G, D'Arrigo G, Gesualdo L. Group E-EIW: renal biopsy in patients with diabetes: a pooled meta-analysis of 48 studies. Nephrol Dial Transplant. 2017;32:97–110.
3. Plantinga LC, Crews DC, Coresh J, Miller ER 3rd, Saran R, Yee J, Hedgeman E, Pavkov M, Eberhardt MS, Williams DE, Powe NR. Prevalence of chronic kidney disease in US adults with undiagnosed diabetes or prediabetes. Clin J Am Soc Nephrol. 2010;5:673–82.
4. Fioretto P, Caramori ML, Mauer M. The kidney in diabetes: dynamic pathways of injury and repair. The Camillo Golgi Lecture 2007. Diabetologia. 2008;51:1347–55.
5. Alicic RZ, Rooney MT, Tuttle KR. Diabetic kidney disease: challenges, progress, and possibilities. Clin J Am Soc Nephrol. 2017;12(12):2032–45.
6. Chan JC, Malik V, Jia W, Kadowaki T, Yajnik CS, Yoon KH, Hu FB. Diabetes in Asia: epidemiology, risk factors, and pathophysiology. JAMA. 2009;301:2129–40.
7. Mise K, Hoshino J, Ubara Y, Sumida K, Hiramatsu R, Hasegawa E, Yamanouchi M, Hayami N, Suwabe T, Sawa N, Fujii T, Ohashi K, Hara S, Takaichi K. Renal prognosis a long time after renal biopsy on patients with diabetic nephropathy. Nephrol Dial Transplant. 2014;29:109–18.

8. Lewis EJ, Hunsicker LG, Bain RP, Rohde RD. The effect of angiotensin-converting-enzyme inhibition on diabetic nephropathy. The Collaborative Study Group. N Engl J Med. 1993;329:1456–62.
9. Brenner BM, Cooper ME, de Zeeuw D, Keane WF, Mitch WE, Parving HH, Remuzzi G, Snapinn SM, Zhang Z, Shahinfar S. Effects of losartan on renal and cardiovascular outcomes in patients with type 2 diabetes and nephropathy. N Engl J Med. 2001;345:861–9.
10. Wanner C, Inzucchi SE, Lachin JM, Fitchett D, von Eynatten M, Mattheus M, Johansen OE, Woerle HJ, Broedl UC, Zinman B, EMPA-REG OUTCOME Investigators. Empagliflozin and progression of kidney disease in type 2 diabetes. N Engl J Med. 2016;375:323–34.
11. Mann JFE, Orsted DD, Brown-Frandsen K, Marso SP, Poulter NR, Rasmussen S, Tornoe K, Zinman B, Buse JB, Leader Steering Committee and Investigators. Liraglutide and renal outcomes in type 2 diabetes. N Engl J Med. 2017;377:839–48.
12. Furuichi K, Shimizu M, Yuzawa Y, Hara A, Toyama T, Kitamura H, Suzuki Y, Sato H, Uesugi N, Ubara Y, Hoshino J, Hisano S, Ueda Y, Nishi S, Yokoyama H, Nishino T, Kohagura K, Ogawa D, Mise K, Shibagaki Y, Kimura K, Haneda M, Makino H, Matsuo S, Wada T, Research Group of Diabetic Nephropathy and Nephrosclerosis tMoH, Labour and Welfare, and the Japan Agency for Medical Research and Development. Nationwide multicenter kidney biopsy study of Japanese patients with hypertensive nephrosclerosis. Clin Exp Nephrol. 2018;22:629–37.
13. Zhuo L, Ren W, Li W, Zou G, Lu J. Evaluation of renal biopsies in type 2 diabetic patients with kidney disease: a clinicopathological study of 216 cases. Int Urol Nephrol. 2013;45:173–9.
14. Nicholas SB. Structural predictors of renal function decline. Clin J Am Soc Nephrol. 2016;11:202–4.
15. Mise K, Hoshino J, Ueno T, Hazue R, Hasegawa J, Sekine A, Sumida K, Hiramatsu R, Hasegawa E, Yamanouchi M, Hayami N, Suwabe T, Sawa N, Fujii T, Hara S, Ohashi K, Takaichi K, Ubara Y. Prognostic value of tubulointerstitial lesions, urinary N-acetyl-beta-d-glucosaminidase, and urinary beta2-microglobulin in patients with type 2 diabetes and biopsy-proven diabetic nephropathy. Clin J Am Soc Nephrol. 2016;11:593–601.
16. Anders HJ, Huber TB, Isermann B, Schiffer M. CKD in diabetes: diabetic kidney disease versus nondiabetic kidney disease. Nat Rev Nephrol. 2018;14:361–77.
17. Wang J, Han Q, Zhao L, Zhang J, Wang Y, Wu Y, Wang T, Zhang R, Grung P, Xu H, Liu F. Identification of clinical predictors of diabetic nephropathy and non-diabetic renal disease in Chinese patients with type 2 diabetes, with reference to disease course and outcome. Acta Diabetol. 2019;56:939–46.
18. Hsieh JT, Chang FP, Yang AH, Tarng DC, Yang CY. Timing of kidney biopsy in type 2 diabetic patients: a stepwise approach. BMC Nephrol. 2020;21:131.
19. Tan J, Zwi LJ, Collins JF, Marshall MR, Cundy T. Presentation, pathology and prognosis of renal disease in type 2 diabetes. BMJ Open Diabetes Res Care. 2017;5:e000412.
20. Oh SW, Kim S, Na KY, Chae DW, Kim S, Jin DC, Chin HJ. Clinical implications of pathologic diagnosis and classification for diabetic nephropathy. Diabetes Res Clin Pract. 2012;97:418–24.
21. Chang TI, Park JT, Kim JK, Kim SJ, Oh HJ, Yoo DE, Han SH, Yoo TH, Kang SW. Renal outcomes in patients with type 2 diabetes with or without coexisting non-diabetic renal disease. Diabetes Res Clin Pract. 2011;92:198–204.
22. Sharma SG, Bomback AS, Radhakrishnan J, Herlitz LC, Stokes MB, Markowitz GS, D'Agati VD. The modern spectrum of renal biopsy findings in patients with diabetes. Clin J Am Soc Nephrol. 2013;8:1718–24.
23. Tone A, Shikata K, Matsuda M, Usui H, Okada S, Ogawa D, Wada J, Makino H. Clinical features of non-diabetic renal diseases in patients with type 2 diabetes. Diabetes Res Clin Pract. 2005;69:237–42.
24. Zhou J, Chen X, Xie Y, Li J, Yamanaka N, Tong X. A differential diagnostic model of diabetic nephropathy and non-diabetic renal diseases. Nephrol Dial Transplant. 2008;23:1940–5.

25. Chong YB, Keng TC, Tan LP, Ng KP, Kong WY, Wong CM, Cheah PL, Looi LM, Tan SY. Clinical predictors of non-diabetic renal disease and role of renal biopsy in diabetic patients with renal involvement: a single centre review. Ren Fail. 2012;34:323–8.
26. Fong DS, Aiello L, Gardner TW, King GL, Blankenship G, Cavallerano JD, Ferris FL 3rd, Klein R. Retinopathy in diabetes. Diabetes Care. 2004;27(Suppl 1):S84–7.
27. Zhang L, Chen B, Tang L. Metabolic memory: mechanisms and implications for diabetic retinopathy. Diabetes Res Clin Pract. 2012;96:286–93.
28. Shimizu M, Furuichi K, Toyama T, Kitajima S, Hara A, Kitagawa K, Iwata Y, Sakai N, Takamura T, Yoshimura M, Yokoyama H, Kaneko S, Wada T. Long-term outcomes of Japanese type 2 diabetic patients with biopsy-proven diabetic nephropathy. Diabetes Care. 2013;36:3655–62.
29. Yamanouchi M, Mori M, Hoshino J, Kinowaki K, Fujii T, Ohashi K, Furuichi K, Wada T, Ubara Y. Retinopathy progression and the risk of end-stage kidney disease: results from a longitudinal Japanese cohort of 232 patients with type 2 diabetes and biopsy-proven diabetic kidney disease. BMJ Open Diabetes Res Care. 2019;7:e000726.
30. Suzuki D, Takano H, Toyoda M, Umezono T, Uehara G, Sakai T, Zhang SY, Mori Y, Yagame M, Endoh M, Sakai H. Evaluation of renal biopsy samples of patients with diabetic nephropathy. Intern Med. 2001;40:1077–84.
31. Jiang S, Wang Y, Zhang Z, Dai P, Yang Y, Li W. Accuracy of hematuria for predicting non-diabetic renal disease in patients with diabetes and kidney disease: a systematic review and meta-analysis. Diabetes Res Clin Pract. 2018;143:288–300.
32. Bi H, Chen N, Ling G, Yuan S, Huang G, Liu R. Nondiabetic renal disease in type 2 diabetic patients: a review of our experience in 220 cases. Ren Fail. 2011;33:26–30.
33. Mise K, Hoshino J, Ueno T, Hazue R, Sumida K, Hiramatsu R, Hasegawa E, Yamanouchi M, Hayami N, Suwabe T, Sawa N, Fujii T, Hara S, Ohashi K, Takaichi K, Ubara Y. Clinical and pathological predictors of estimated GFR decline in patients with type 2 diabetes and overt proteinuric diabetic nephropathy. Diabetes Metab Res Rev. 2015;31:572–81.
34. Mise K, Hoshino J, Ueno T, Sumida K, Hiramatsu R, Hasegawa E, Yamanouchi M, Hayami N, Suwabe T, Sawa N, Fujii T, Hara S, Ohashi K, Takaichi K, Ubara Y. Clinical implications of linear immunofluorescent staining for immunoglobulin G in patients with diabetic nephropathy. Diabetes Res Clin Pract. 2014;106:522–30.

Chapter 13
Experimental Animal Models of Diabetic Kidney Disease

Shinya Nagasaka and Akira Shimizu

13.1 Pathological Lesions of Diabetic Nephropathy

In humans, the clinical characterizations of diabetic kidney disease (DKD) are the development of microalbuminuria subsequently progressing to macroalbuminuria, nephrotic syndrome, and progressive decline in renal function [1, 2]. The characteristic histological features in human diabetic nephropathy (DN) include glomerular hypertrophy, glomerular basement membrane (GBM) thickening by electron microscopy without immune deposits, mesangial matrix expansion and sclerosis (diffuse diabetic glomerulosclerosis) with or without the formation of nodular diabetic glomerulosclerosis (Kimmelstiel-Wilson lesions), exudative lesions (known as fibrin cap, capsular drop, and arteriolar hyalinosis of afferent and efferent arterioles), and tubulointerstitial lesions including Armanni-Ebstein lesions and paratubular basement membrane (BM) insudative lesions [2, 3].

In 2010, the pathological classification of DN in type 1 and type 2 diabetes mellitus (DM) was reported by the Renal Pathology Society [4]. It was divided into four classes: class I, thickening of the GBM and nonspecific changes by light microscopy; class II, mild (IIa) or severe (IIb) mesangial expansion (diffuse lesions); class III, nodular sclerosis (Kimmelstiel-Wilson lesions) in at least one glomerulus; and class IV, advanced diabetic glomerulosclerosis observed as a global glomerular sclerosis in more than 50% of the glomeruli.

In Japan, the pathological evaluation factors for the standardization of the pathological diagnosis of DN and the definition of the pathological findings have been established [5]. The Japanese pathological classification of DN is scored for glomerular lesions, such as diffuse lesions (mesangial expansion), nodular lesions (nodular sclerosis), subendothelial space widening (double contour of the GBM), exudative lesions, mesangiolysis/microaneurysm, perihilar neovascularization

S. Nagasaka · A. Shimizu (✉)
Department of Analytic Human Pathology, Nippon Medical School, Tokyo, Japan
e-mail: ashimizu@nms.ac.jp

T. Wada et al. (eds.), *Diabetic Kidney Disease*,
https://doi.org/10.1007/978-981-15-9301-7_13

(polar vasculosis), global glomerulosclerosis/collapsed or ischemic glomerulopathy, segmental glomerulosclerosis, glomerulomegaly, interstitial lesions including interstitial fibrosis and tubular atrophy, interstitial inflammation, and vascular lesions such as arteriolar hyalinosis and intimal thickening.

In human DKD, podocyte loss or dysfunction has also been observed in the progression of DN with albuminuria, proteinuria, and nephrotic syndrome, and detachment of podocytes from the GBM can be traced in the urine [6–8]. The podocyte injury may be associated with the generation of reactive oxygen species (ROS) by NADPH oxidase in the podocytes [6, 9].

In tubulointerstitial lesions, tubular hypertrophy, thickening of the tubular BM, tubular atrophy, inflammatory cell infiltration, and interstitial fibrosis are developed in DN [6, 10, 11]. In addition, Armanni-Ebstein lesions and paratubular BM insudative lesions are known as the characteristic histological findings of DN.

As arteriolar hyalinosis of afferent and efferent arterioles, arteries and arterioles in the kidney can also be affected by the DM condition, and vascular dysfunction including the enhancement of vascular permeability and the generation of ROS leads to renal and vascular diseases in DN [6, 12].

These glomerular, tubulointerstitial, and vascular lesions cooperatively play important roles in the progression of DKD as well as decline in renal function. Therefore, animal models of DN should reflect these characteristic pathological features in the glomeruli, tubulointerstitium, and vasculatures.

13.2 Animal Models of DKD

For many diseases, animal models have been powerful tools to investigate the pathogenesis and for the development of novel therapies. In the research studies into human DKD, there are numerous models of spontaneous and acquired (e.g., streptozotocin [STZ] injection) DM [13–16]. Using animal models of DKD enables us to introduce the pathogenesis and time course of the development of DN. However, a rodent model that completely develops all of both the clinical and pathological features of human DKD is not currently available. Each rodent model of DM has their own limitations for the investigation of type 1 and type 2 DM. Therefore, each experimental study should select the appropriate model of DM for each purpose of the study.

13.2.1 Type 1 DM Models

13.2.1.1 STZ-Injected Rodent Models

The STZ-induced rodent model is the most widely used experimental model for type 1 DM research. STZ is toxic to the pancreatic β-cells, resulting in absolute insulin deficiency. However, when administered at high doses (150–200 mg/Kg), STZ may also injure other organs, including the kidney [17]. Therefore, it is necessary to minimize the nonspecific toxicity of STZ to organs other than the pancreatic β-cells. To accomplish this, multiple injections of low doses of STZ are required to induce DM in rodent animals [18].

13.2.1.2 STZ-Injected Rat Models

It is known that rats are more susceptible to STZ-induced DM than mice and are more relevant to human diseases in many characteristics, such as genetics and pathophysiology [19]. Recently, advanced techniques have enabled the manipulation of targeted genes in rats (e.g., knockout and transgenic rats) [20]. However, recapitulating the murine gene manipulation techniques in rats requires several years and includes the additional costs of generating transgenic rodents. Although it is difficult to cause gene modification in STZ-injected rat models, they are widely used in DKD studies because hyperglycemia can be easily induced.

DM is usually induced in male Sprague-Dawley (SD), Wistar-Kyoto (WKY), or other rats weighing 170–250 g by a single intravenous injection of STZ (40–70 mg/kg body weight) [1, 21, 22]. One week after STZ injection, the rats should be assessed for hyperglycemia. Those with fasting blood glucose of over 15 mmol/L (280 mg/dL), which is usually approximately 90% in injected rats, typically develop type 1 DM within 2–3 weeks. The STZ-induced DM rats have an increase in the mesangial matrix and an accumulation of type IV collagen in the glomeruli compared to the control rats [2]. However, some characteristic pathological findings that are observed in human DN, such as exudative lesions and nodular lesions in the glomeruli, or tubulointerstitial lesions, do not develop. STZ-injected rat model is useful for the assessment of the early morphological and physiological changes of DN.

13.2.1.3 STZ-Injected Mouse Models

Mice are relatively cheap to breed and house, and it is comparatively easy to manipulate their genome; thus, they are the most commonly used species in basic and preclinical research. C57BL/6 mice are the most commonly used strain and many genetic modifications can be conducted [19]. The STZ-induced DM mouse model is widely used for both basic and preclinical research, including the study of DM complications. Based on the AMDCC (Animal Models of Diabetic Complications Consortium) protocol, this method consists of daily intraperitoneal injections of STZ (40–50 mg/kg) for 5 consecutive days [2]. At the late stage of the disease, STZ-induced DM mice may exhibit significant weight loss, possibly due to insulin deficiency and severe hyperglycemia, as well as the volume depletion associated with osmotic diuresis. However, the C57BL/6 strain is relatively resistant to the development of DN associated with moderate albuminuria [23]. Some renal pathological lesions, including glomerular hypertrophy, a thickening of the GBM, and a slight expansion of the mesangial matrix, were observed in the STZ-induced DM model in the C57BL/6 strain at the later stage [23, 24]. This can be a useful model for elucidating the characteristics of early phase of DN. STZ-induced DM C57BL/6 mice are usually less susceptible to diabetic kidney injury than other strains [13, 23, 24], and it is possible that genetic mutations by backcrossing onto a more susceptible strain such as FVB and DBA/2 mice are required.

13.2.1.4 STZ-DBA/2 Mice

STZ-induced DM DBA/2 mice develop more marked albuminuria at 5 weeks after the induction of DM and further pronounced albuminuria after 25 weeks compared to C57BL/6 mice [23]. They also exhibit the pathological features of human DN, such as thickening of the GBM, serious mesangial matrix expansion, nodular glomerulosclerosis, and arteriolar hyalinosis in the later phase after induction of DM [23]. In addition, some renal tubular damage including enlargement of the tubules and tubular atrophy are also observed in this strain, although no obvious tubulointerstitial fibrosis has been observed [24]. DBA/2 mice are highly susceptible to renal injury for STZ-induced DN compared to the C57BL/6 strain, and this strain can be useful as a model of DN in type 1 DM [2].

13.2.1.5 STZ-eNOS KO Mice

Functional deficiency of eNOS has been observed in DM patients [25] and is associated with impaired vascular nitric oxide (NO) production. The polymorphisms of the eNOS gene located on human chromosome 7 are involved in DM vasculopathies [26–30]. In experimental DM models, eNOS knockout (eNOS KO) mice exhibit important pathogenic mechanisms related to human DKD, such as endothelial dysfunction and hypertension [25]. Compared to STZ-induced DM WT mice, diabetic eNOS KO mice exhibit many typical physiological and pathological findings of human DN, including decreased glomerular filtration rate (GFR) with the massive and early onset of albuminuria, and thickening of the GBM, mesangial expansion, mesangiolysis, Kimmelstiel-Wilson nodular lesions in glomeruli, and arteriolar hyalinosis [31, 32]. Importantly, these features in eNOS KO mice are observed even in the DN-resistant C57BL6 strain [31, 32]. Among the mouse models of type 1 DM, the STZ-injected C57BL/6 eNOS KO mouse is the most useful for studying the features of advanced DN [33], and this model enables the study of the genomic/molecular and pathogenic mechanisms of progressive DKD by combining with other knockout/transgenic mice that have already been established or will be in the future.

13.2.1.6 Akita (Ins2+/C96Y) Mice

The Akita mouse is one of the first described mouse models to spontaneously develop type 1 DM [34–36]. Akita mice have a single nucleotide substitution in the insulin 2 gene (Ins2+/C96Y), originally identified as a spontaneous mutation in a colony of the C57BL/6 mice strain. This mutation causes abnormal folding of the insulin protein, endoplasmic reticulum stress, nonspecific dysfunction of the secretory pathways, and toxic injury to the pancreatic β-cells, resulting in the development of type 1 DM [2, 35, 37]. Akita mice show severe irreversible hyperglycemia and hypoinsulinemia, which are central features of this model [9, 38]. These mice are commercially available from Jackson Laboratories. On the C57BL/6 background, hyperglycemia is considerably worse in the male mice than the females. Akita DM mice of the C57BL/6 strain develop modest structural changes that are observed in human DN, including thickening of the GBM, increase in the mesangial matrix, mesangiolysis, nodular mesangial sclerosis, and podocyte loss [9, 39]. Furthermore, these mice have not only these pathophysiological features, which are replicates of DN, but also increased oxidative stress, inflammation, and premature senescence, which play important roles in the pathogenesis and development of DN [40–46]. Notably, Akita mice with a C57BL/6 genetic background have significant diffuse granular mesangial deposits of IgA at 20 weeks of age [38]. Compared to controls, male Akita DM mice, but not female mice, develop decreased renal function associated with increased serum IgA after 30 weeks of age [2]. The significance of these findings concerning mesangial deposition of IgA is uncertain [47], but Akita Ins2+/C96Y mice with a C57BL/6 genetic background are unique mouse models of DKD in type 1 DM.

13.2.1.7 OVE26 Mice

The OVE26 mouse is another transgenic diabetic mouse model that exhibits most of the morphological characteristics of human DN with chronic hyperglycemia [48–51]. OVE26 mice with an FVB background overexpress calmodulin in the pancreatic β-cells, leading to the deficient production of insulin within the first week of life and resulting in the development of type 1 DM, as these pancreatic β-cells rapidly disappear due to apoptosis caused by oxidative stress in the endoplasmic reticulum [52, 53]. However, in heterozygotes OVE26 mice, pancreatic β-cells slightly retained, and these mice can survive over 1 year without insulin treatment [54–57]. OVE26 mice are therefore well suited for a long-term assessment of DKD because of their long life spans (>450 days) [54]. OVE26 mice exhibit histological changes that are comparatively similar to those of human DN, including enlarged glomeruli, thickening of the GBM, increased mesangial matrix with diffuse expansion at 6 months of age [49], and nodular lesions at 7-month-old mice [48, 51, 58]. The development of modest interstitial fibrosis requires 5–8 months, and a 20% decline in the GFR is not observed until 9 months of age [48]. When the transgene is introduced into the C57BL/6 or DBA/2 mouse strains, albuminuria, increased mesangial matrix, and interstitial fibrosis are all diminished [54]. Oxidative stress and inflammation are induced in these mouse kidneys, which are related to the pathogenesis and progression of DKD [46]. Altogether, OVE26 DM mice are particularly valuable as they possess numerous features of human DKD [48, 49, 59, 60] and allow us to conduct experiments on DKD treatments.

13.2.2 Type 2 Diabetes Models

13.2.2.1 Ob/Ob (BTBR) Mice

It was recently reported that the interesting but relatively unfamiliar mouse strain, black and tan brachyuric (BTBR), may be a potentially useful strain for a model of DKD [16, 61, 62]. BTBR strain mice are naturally insulin-resistant, and when the ob/ob leptin-deficient mutation is introduced into this strain, the mice exhibit sustained hyperglycemia from an early age and develop pathological features very closely resembling human DN in type 2 DM [33, 61–63]. In the ob/ob (BTBR) mice, podocyte loss and albuminuria are detectable by 8 weeks of age, mesangial expansion is identifiable by 10 weeks of age [61], and by 18 weeks of age, increased proteinuria, thickening of the GBM, extensive mesangial matrix expansion, mesangiolysis and sclerosis, focal nodular glomerulosclerosis, and persistent podocyte loss in glomeruli are developed with mild interstitial fibrosis and arteriolar hyalinosis [33, 61, 62, 64]. The reversibility of physiological and pathological findings by the continuous infusion of leptin is particularly advantageous in this ob/ob (BTBR) mouse model [65]. The mortality rate of these mice increases over 24 weeks of age, which makes it difficult to use them as a long-term DKD model. Similar to other leptin-deficient mice, ob/ob (BTBR) mice have poor fertility, making it difficult to prepare sufficient numbers for pathological studies. While ob/ob (BTBR) mice have these limitations for DKD study, the advantages of these mice as a model of human DKD compared to other DKD model animals are the comparatively rapid development of DKD and the reversibility of functional and pathological changes.

13.2.2.2 Db/Db Mice

The db/db mouse model that lacks leptin receptors is currently the most widely used mouse model for studying the pathology of human DN in type 2 DM settings [2, 13, 66]. The db gene encodes for a point mutation (G to T) in the leptin receptor gene (LepRdb/db), resulting in abnormal splicing and defective signaling for the adipocyte-derived hormone leptin [13, 67–69]. This LepRdb/db mutation with a C57BLKS background was originally identified in 1966 in Jackson Laboratories in an obese mouse [69] and was modified to share part of the genetic background with the DBA/2 strain [70]. The lack of leptin signaling in the hypothalamus in db/db mice leads to the development of hyperphagia, obesity, hyperlipidemia, hyperinsulinemia, insulin resistance, and type 2 DM. Male db/db mice exhibit more severe DM than female mice. Hyperinsulinemia is exhibited by 10 days of age, and blood glucose levels are increased with aging [71]. Pathological features of DN are observed in db/db mice such as an increase in GBM thickening [72–74], podocyte loss [9, 13, 75–77], and diffuse mesangial expansion [78–81] with increased type IV collagen, fibronectin, and laminin [75, 82–85] at 20–24 weeks, and they progressed by 18–20 months. db/db mice with a C57BLKS background are a good model of the early pathological changes that are associated with human DN.

13.2.2.3 Db/Db eNOS KO Mice

In contrast to db/db mice exhibiting mild changes in the DKD, db/db eNOS KO mice with a C57BLKS background, which lack both eNOS and leptin receptor genes, develop more advanced DKD in type 2 DM [86, 87]. Hyperglycemia is first detected at 6–8 weeks age, and full-blown renal dysfunction and kidney injury develop with significant albuminemia by 16–20 weeks of age. In db/db eNOS KO mice, extensive mesangial matrix expansion, thickening of the GBM, mesangiolysis, focal segmental and early nodular glomerulosclerosis in glomeruli are developed with tubulointerstitial lesions and arteriolar hyalinosis [86–88] (Fig. 13.1). Furthermore, db/db eNOS KO mice exhibit a 50% reduction in the GFR at 26 weeks of age compared to db/db eNOS WT mice, as confirmed by increased serum creatinine levels [87]. In db/db eNOS KO mice, similar to other spontaneous DM mouse models, these mice have difficulty breeding because of their combined mutations.

13.2.2.4 KK-Ay Mice

The KK/Ta mouse, a model of DKD in type 2 DM, was developed from Japanese native mice in 1957; however, this mouse has relatively weak lesions [89]. The KK-Ay mouse was established by transferring the yellow obese gene (Ay allele) into a KK/Ta mouse in 1969 [2, 89]. KK-Ay mice exhibit obesity, hyperglycemia, and albuminuria by 16 weeks of age [90]. These mice are widely used as an experimental model for type 2 DM [2, 89–91]. At 16 weeks of age, in KK-Ay mice, renal morphological changes, including diffuse and moderate to severe mesangial matrix expansion and nodular glomerulosclerosis in glomeruli, are developed [90, 91]. The reduced podocytes associated with the progression of glomerular lesions are also observed in KK-Ay mice [89]. In addition, oxidative stress and inflammation have also been observed in the kidneys of KK-Ay mice consistent with human DKD [90, 92].

13.2.2.5 ZDF Rats

Zucker diabetic fatty (ZDF) rats are derived from male Zucker fatty rats, which have a homozygous missense mutation (fatty, fa) in the leptin receptor gene and develop obesity without DM [2, 93–95]. However, ZDF rats develop progressive insulin resistance and glucose intolerance at 3–8 weeks of age and subsequently exhibit DM [2]. ZDF rats are widely used as a model of type 2 DM. Albuminuria

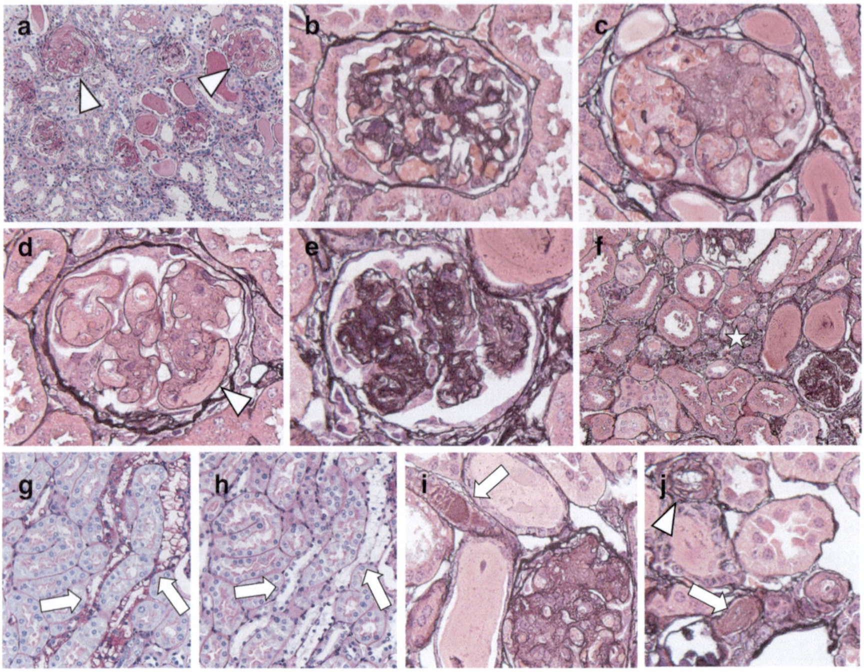

Fig. 13.1 Light microscopic findings of diabetic nephropathy in db/db eNOS KO mouse model at 24 weeks old. (**a**) In diabetic nephropathy in db/db eNOS KO mice, the glomeruli show various glomerular lesions with glomerular hypertrophy (arrowhead). The tubules also show the dilation with protein casts (periodic acid-Schiff [PAS] stain, ×200). (**b**) This glomerulus shows diffuse mesangial expansion with accumulation of mesangial matrix, indicating the development of diffuse lesion of diabetic nephropathy (periodic acid-methenamine silver [PAM] stain, ×600). (**c**) This glomerulus shows irregular large capillary lumens without mesangial areas, indicating the development of diffuse and the early phase of mesangiolysis of diabetic nephropathy (PAM stain, ×600). (**d**) This glomerulus shows the accumulation of extracellular matrix in mesangiolytic areas with exudative lesions, namely, fibrin (hyaline) cap (arrowhead) (PAM stain, ×600). (**e**) The multiple nodular glomerulosclerosis, namely, Kimmelstiel-Wilson lesions, is noted in this glomerulus (PAM stain, ×600). (**f**) In tubulointerstitium, the dilatation of renal tubules with protein casts and the atrophy of renal tubules (star) are evident with interstitial fibrosis. The glomeruli with diffuse and/or nodular glomerulosclerosis are also seen (PAM stain, ×300). (**g**, **h**) The serial sections with PAS stain (**g**) and PAS diastase stain (**h**) show the vacuolization and PAS-positive glycogen accumulation within the cytoplasm of tubular epithelial cells, namely, Armanni-Ebstein lesions in tubules (arrows) (×400). (**i**, **j**) Arteriolar hyalinosis (arrow in **i** and **j**) and thickening of arterial intima (arrowhead in **j**) develop in small arterioles (PAM stain, ×600)

progressively increases with aging [96, 97], and the pathological changes, including diffuse mesangial matrix expansion, and tubulointerstitial fibrosis and tubular atrophy are observed in the kidneys of ZDF rats between 22 and 39 weeks of age [98]. However, these rats do not exhibit mesangiolysis or nodular glomerulosclerosis, which are representative findings in advanced human DN.

13.2.2.6 OLETF Rats

The Otsuka Long-Evans Tokushima Fatty (OLETF) rat is a model of spontaneously developing type 2 DM [2, 99]. These rats exhibit many pathophysiological and morphological characteristics of human DKD in type 2 DM. In male OLETF rats, impaired glucose tolerance and increased plasma glucose levels are initiated from 8 and 18 weeks of age. OLETF rats develop DM by 25 weeks of age and exhibit early phases of the disease, such as hyperglycemia and hyperinsulinemia [100]. Thereafter, they eventually develop hypoinsulinemia at over 40 weeks of age as a result of the degradation of pancreatic β-cells [2, 101]. OLETF male rats start exhibiting higher albuminuria from 10 weeks of age, and thereafter this progressively increases to ~200 mg/days at 36 weeks of age [102]. At 40 weeks of age, thickening of the GBM, moderate mesangial matrix expansion, and nodular glomerulosclerosis in glomeruli are observed with tubulointerstitial lesions, such as inflammatory cell infiltration and fibrosis [99]. Thus, male OLETF rats may be a useful model for investigating both glomerular and tubulointerstitial injuries in advanced DN of type 2 DM.

13.2.2.7 Goto-Kakizaki (GK) Rats

The Goto-Kakizaki (GK) rat is a spontaneous model of type 2 diabetes without obesity, which was originally established by repetitive inbreeding of glucose intolerant Wistar rats [103]. GK rats exhibit glucose intolerance as early as 2 weeks of age due to impaired insulin secretion rather than insulin tolerance and subsequently develop type 2 DM as confirmed by the elevation of plasma glucose and insulin levels by 12 weeks of age [2, 93, 104, 105]. Several histological changes in the kidney have been reported, including glomerular hypertrophy, thickening of the GBM, mild to moderate mesangial matrix expansion, oxidative stress, and inflammation [2, 106–108]. However, GK rats are relatively resistant to kidney injury in DM [105], and they do not develop progressive DN renal injuries, such as massive proteinuria and renal dysfunction, as well as renal pathology including remarkable mesangial matrix expansion, nodular sclerosis, global glomerulosclerosis, and tubulointerstitial fibrosis [2, 109].

13.2.2.8 WBN/Kob-Leprfa Rats

The male WBN/Kob rat is another spontaneous DM model that commonly develops chronic pancreatitis by 3 months of age and subsequently develops DM (characterized by hyperglycemia, hypoinsulinemia, and glycosuria) by 9 months of age [110, 111]. WBN/Kob-Leprfa rats are introduced with the leptin receptor fatty mutation (Leprfa) leading to leptin receptor deficiency in WBN/Kob rats. Homozygous animals (fa/fa) commonly develop not only pancreatitis at 7–9 weeks of age, but also obesity, insulin resistance, and hyperinsulinemia, resulting in type 2 DM at 3–4 months [110]. A few pathological features in the kidney of WBN/Kob-Leprfa rats have been reported, including modest mesangial matrix expansion in the glomeruli, glycogenotic tubules known as Armanni-Ebstein lesions, tubular dilation with protein casts, and inflammatory cell infiltration into the renal cortex [112]. WBN/Kob-Leprfa rats may be a useful model of human type 2 DM because they develop salt-sensitive hypertension and non-insulin-dependent DM. However, the pathological features of the renal lesions have not been fully elucidated and further analysis is necessary.

13.3 Conclusion

Despite many efforts thus far to establish rodent models of DKD that replicate the pathophysiology and morphological features of human DN in type 1 and type 2 DM as close as possible, ideal models have not yet been developed. However, currently available models of DM exhibit physiological findings including albuminuria, proteinuria, and renal dysfunction, as well as characteristic renal pathological lesions of DN such as GBM thickening, diffuse glomerular lesion, nodular glomerular lesion, tubulointerstitial lesions, and arteriolar hyalinosis. Therefore, these rodent models may be helpful for understanding the pathophysiological features and the pathogenesis of onset and progression of DN. When using these rodent models, it is necessary to be aware that not all of the morphological abnormalities of human DKD can be reproduced. In addition, genetic backgrounds and breeding difficulty are also considered in the assessment of DKD using animal models. Therefore, it is important to understand the limitations and features of each rodent model, and researchers need to select the appropriate animal model according to the research subject (Table 13.1).

Table 13.1 Rodent models of diabetic kidney disease (DKD)

Model	Pathological features	Notices	Reference(s)
Type 1 DKD			
STZ-injected rat (SD rat or WKY rat)	Increased mesangial matrix Accumulation of type IV collagen	Weak mesangial matrix accumulation No nodular glomerulosclerosis Weak tubulointerstitial fibrosis	[1, 2, 21, 22]
STZ-C57BL/6 mice	Glomerular hypertrophy Thickening of GBM Slight expansion of mesangial matrix Dilatation of tubules and tubular atrophy	Relatively resistant to the development of DKD	[23, 24]

Table 13.1 (continued)

Model	Pathological features	Notices	Reference(s)
STZ-DBA/2 mice	Thickening of GBM Serious mesangial matrix expansion Nodular glomerulosclerosis Dilatation of tubules and tubular atrophy Arteriolar hyalinosis	Highly susceptible to STZ-induced renal injury No obvious tubulointerstitial fibrosis	[23, 24]
STZ-eNOS KO mice (C57BL/6 background)	Thickening of GBM Mesangial matrix expansion Mesangiolysis Nodular glomerulosclerosis Arteriolar hyalinosis	Weak tubulointerstitial fibrosis	[25, 31, 32]
Akita (Ins2+/C96Y) mice	Thickening of GBM Increased mesangial matrix Mesangiolysis Nodular glomerulosclerosis Podocyte loss Tubulointerstitial fibrosis	Irreversible hyperglycemia and hypoinsulinemia Granular mesangial deposit of IgA	[9, 38–46]
OVE26 mice	Enlarged glomeruli Thickening of GBM Mesangial matrix expansion Nodular glomerulosclerosis Podocyte loss Tubulointerstitial fibrosis Arteriolar hyalinosis	Long life (>450 days) Low viability	[48–51, 54, 58]
Type 2 DKD			
Ob/ob (BTBR) mice	Thickening of GBM Mesangial matrix expansion Mesangiolysis and sclerosis Nodular glomerulosclerosis (focal) Podocyte loss Arteriolar hyalinosis	Mild interstitial fibrosis Reversibility of morphological changes Moderate level of albuminuria No significant change in serum creatinine High mortality rate over 24 weeks of age Poor fertility	[33, 61–65]
Db/db mice	Thickening of GBM Diffuse mesangial expansion Podocyte loss	Leptin receptor gene point mutation (G to T) C57BLKS background No significant increase of albuminuria	[2, 13, 66–69, 72–81]
Db/db eNOS KO mice	Thickening of GBM Mesangial matrix expansion Mesangiolysis Nodular glomerulosclerosis (focal) Arteriolar hyalinosis Tubulointerstitial lesions	Decreased GFR Difficulty in breeding	[86–88]

(continued)

Table 13.1 (continued)

Model	Pathological features	Notices	Reference(s)
KK-Ay mice	Diffuse mesangial matrix expansion Segmental sclerosis Nodular glomerulosclerosis Podocyte loss	Oxidative stress Inflammation No tubulointerstitial fibrosis	[89–92]
ZDF rats	Mesangial matrix expansion Tubulointerstitial fibrosis	No nodular glomerulosclerosis No mesangiolysis Insulin resistance and glucose tolerance No atherosclerosis	[96–98]
OLETF rats	Thickening of GBM Mesangial matrix expansion Nodular glomerulosclerosis Tubulointerstitial fibrosis	Delayed onsetIncreased GFR Hypoinsulinemia	[2, 99–102]
Goto-Kakizaki (GK) rats	Glomerular hypertrophy Thickening of GBM Mesangial matrix expansion (mild) Thickening of arterial intima	No nodular glomerulosclerosis No tubulointerstitial fibrosis No atherosclerosis Weak proteinuria No renal dysfunction	[2, 105–109]
WBN/Kob-Lepr^{fa} rats	Insufficient analysis of renal pathology Mesangial matrix expansion Armanni-Ebstein lesions	Insulin resistance Hyperinsulinemia Pancreatitis Salt-sensitive hypertension	[110, 112]

STZ streptozotocin, *GBM* glomerular basement membrane, *eNOS* endothelial nitric oxide synthase, *GFR* glomerular filtration rate

References

1. Tesch GH, Allen TJ. Rodent models of streptozotocin-induced diabetic nephropathy. Nephrology (Carlton). 2007;12(3):261–6. https://doi.org/10.1111/j.1440-1797.2007.00796.x.
2. Kitada M, Ogura Y, Koya D. Rodent models of diabetic nephropathy: their utility and limitations. Int J Nephrol Renovasc Dis. 2016;9:279–90. https://doi.org/10.2147/IJNRD.S103784.
3. Mise K, Yamaguchi Y, Hoshino J, Ueno T, Sekine A, Sumida K, et al. Paratubular basement membrane insudative lesions predict renal prognosis in patients with type 2 diabetes and biopsy-proven diabetic nephropathy. PLoS One. 2017;12(8):e0183190. https://doi.org/10.1371/journal.pone.0183190.
4. Tervaert TW, Mooyaart AL, Amann K, Cohen AH, Cook HT, Drachenberg CB, et al. Pathologic classification of diabetic nephropathy. J Am Soc Nephrol. 2010;21(4):556–63. https://doi.org/10.1681/ASN.2010010010.
5. Furuichi K, Yuzawa Y, Shimizu M, Hara A, Toyama T, Kitamura H, et al. Nationwide multicentre kidney biopsy study of Japanese patients with type 2 diabetes. Nephrol Dial Transplant. 2018;33(1):138–48. https://doi.org/10.1093/ndt/gfw417.
6. Pourghasem M, Shafi H, Babazadeh Z. Histological changes of kidney in diabetic nephropathy. Caspian J Intern Med. 2015;6(3):120–7.

7. Schiffer M, Bitzer M, Roberts IS, Kopp JB, ten Dijke P, Mundel P, et al. Apoptosis in podocytes induced by TGF-beta and Smad7. J Clin Invest. 2001;108(6):807–16. https://doi.org/10.1172/JCI12367.
8. Nakamura T, Ushiyama C, Suzuki S, Hara M, Shimada N, Ebihara I, et al. Urinary excretion of podocytes in patients with diabetic nephropathy. Nephrol Dial Transplant. 2000;15(9):1379–83.
9. Susztak K, Raff AC, Schiffer M, Bottinger EP. Glucose-induced reactive oxygen species cause apoptosis of podocytes and podocyte depletion at the onset of diabetic nephropathy. Diabetes. 2006;55(1):225–33.
10. An Y, Xu F, Le W, Ge Y, Zhou M, Chen H, et al. Renal histologic changes and the outcome in patients with diabetic nephropathy. Nephrol Dial Transplant. 2015;30(2):257–66. https://doi.org/10.1093/ndt/gfu250.
11. Najafian B, Alpers CE, Fogo AB. Pathology of human diabetic nephropathy. Contrib Nephrol. 2011;170:36–47. https://doi.org/10.1159/000324942.
12. Deen WM, Lazzara MJ, Myers BD. Structural determinants of glomerular permeability. Am J Physiol Renal Physiol. 2001;281(4):F579–96. https://doi.org/10.1152/ajprenal.2001.281.4.F579.
13. Breyer MD, Bottinger E, Brosius FC 3rd, Coffman TM, Harris RC, Heilig CW, et al. Mouse models of diabetic nephropathy. J Am Soc Nephrol. 2005;16(1):27–45. https://doi.org/10.1681/ASN.2004080648.
14. Breyer MD, Qi Z, Tchekneva EE, Harris RC. Insight into the genetics of diabetic nephropathy through the study of mice. Curr Opin Nephrol Hypertens. 2008;17(1):82–6. https://doi.org/10.1097/MNH.0b013e3282f49cc9.
15. Brosius FC 3rd, Alpers CE, Bottinger EP, Breyer MD, Coffman TM, Gurley SB, et al. Mouse models of diabetic nephropathy. J Am Soc Nephrol. 2009;20(12):2503–12. https://doi.org/10.1681/ASN.2009070721.
16. Azushima K, Gurley SB, Coffman TM. Modelling diabetic nephropathy in mice. Nat Rev Nephrol. 2018;14(1):48–56. https://doi.org/10.1038/nrneph.2017.142.
17. Bolzan AD, Bianchi MS. Genotoxicity of streptozotocin. Mutat Res. 2002;512(2–3):121–34.
18. Like AA, Appel MC, Williams RM, Rossini AA. Streptozotocin-induced pancreatic insulitis in mice. Morphologic and physiologic studies. Lab Invest. 1978;38(4):470–86.
19. Betz B, Conway BR. An update on the use of animal models in diabetic nephropathy research. Curr DiabRep. 2016;16(2):18. https://doi.org/10.1007/s11892-015-0706-2.
20. Geurts AM, Cost GJ, Freyvert Y, Zeitler B, Miller JC, Choi VM, et al. Knockout rats via embryo microinjection of zinc-finger nucleases. Science. 2009;325(5939):433. https://doi.org/10.1126/science.1172447.
21. Kitada M, Koya D, Sugimoto T, Isono M, Araki S, Kashiwagi A, et al. Translocation of glomerular p47phox and p67phox by protein kinase C-beta activation is required for oxidative stress in diabetic nephropathy. Diabetes. 2003;52(10):2603–14.
22. Brondum E, Nilsson H, Aalkjaer C. Functional abnormalities in isolated arteries from Goto-Kakizaki and streptozotocin-treated diabetic rat models. Horm Metab Res. 2005;37(Suppl 1):56–60. https://doi.org/10.1055/s-2005-861370.
23. Qi Z, Fujita H, Jin J, Davis LS, Wang Y, Fogo AB, et al. Characterization of susceptibility of inbred mouse strains to diabetic nephropathy. Diabetes. 2005;54(9):2628–37.
24. Sugimoto H, Grahovac G, Zeisberg M, Kalluri R. Renal fibrosis and glomerulosclerosis in a new mouse model of diabetic nephropathy and its regression by bone morphogenic protein-7 and advanced glycation end product inhibitors. Diabetes. 2007;56(7):1825–33. https://doi.org/10.2337/db06-1226.
25. Nakayama T, Sato W, Kosugi T, Zhang L, Campbell-Thompson M, Yoshimura A, et al. Endothelial injury due to eNOS deficiency accelerates the progression of chronic renal disease in the mouse. Am J Physiol Renal Physiol. 2009;296(2):F317–27. https://doi.org/10.1152/ajprenal.90450.2008.

26. Nakayama T, Soma M, Takahashi Y, Izumi Y, Kanmatsuse K, Esumi M. Association analysis of CA repeat polymorphism of the endothelial nitric oxide synthase gene with essential hypertension in Japanese. Clin Genet. 1997;51(1):26–30.
27. Arngrimsson R, Hayward C, Nadaud S, Baldursdottir A, Walker JJ, Liston WA, et al. Evidence for a familial pregnancy-induced hypertension locus in the eNOS-gene region. Am J Hum Genet. 1997;61(2):354–62. https://doi.org/10.1086/514843.
28. Yokoyama K, Tsukada T, Matsuoka H, Hara S, Yamada A, Kawaguchi Y. High accumulation of endothelial nitric oxide synthase (ecNOS): a gene polymorphism in patients with end-stage renal disease. Nephron. 1998;79(3):360–1. https://doi.org/10.1159/000045069.
29. Yoshimura M, Yasue H, Nakayama M, Shimasaki Y, Sumida H, Sugiyama S, et al. A missense Glu298Asp variant in the endothelial nitric oxide synthase gene is associated with coronary spasm in the Japanese. Hum Genet. 1998;103(1):65–9.
30. Miyamoto Y, Saito Y, Kajiyama N, Yoshimura M, Shimasaki Y, Nakayama M, et al. Endothelial nitric oxide synthase gene is positively associated with essential hypertension. Hypertension. 1998;32(1):3–8.
31. Nakagawa T, Sato W, Glushakova O, Heinig M, Clarke T, Campbell-Thompson M, et al. Diabetic endothelial nitric oxide synthase knockout mice develop advanced diabetic nephropathy. J Am Soc Nephrol. 2007;18(2):539–50. https://doi.org/10.1681/ASN.2006050459.
32. Kanetsuna Y, Takahashi K, Nagata M, Gannon MA, Breyer MD, Harris RC, et al. Deficiency of endothelial nitric-oxide synthase confers susceptibility to diabetic nephropathy in nephropathy-resistant inbred mice. Am J Pathol. 2007;170(5):1473–84. https://doi.org/10.2353/ajpath.2007.060481.
33. Yu L, Su Y, Paueksakon P, Cheng H, Chen X, Wang H, et al. Integrin alpha1/Akita double-knockout mice on a Balb/c background develop advanced features of human diabetic nephropathy. Kidney Int. 2012;81(11):1086–97. https://doi.org/10.1038/ki.2011.474.
34. Mathews CE, Langley SH, Leiter EH. New mouse model to study islet transplantation in insulin-dependent diabetes mellitus. Transplantation. 2002;73(8):1333–6.
35. Wang J, Takeuchi T, Tanaka S, Kubo SK, Kayo T, Lu D, et al. A mutation in the insulin 2 gene induces diabetes with severe pancreatic beta-cell dysfunction in the Mody mouse. J Clin Invest. 1999;103(1):27–37. https://doi.org/10.1172/JCI4431.
36. Yoshioka M, Kayo T, Ikeda T, Koizumi A. A novel locus, Mody4, distal to D7Mit189 on chromosome 7 determines early-onset NIDDM in nonobese C57BL/6 (Akita) mutant mice. Diabetes. 1997;46(5):887–94.
37. Ron D. Proteotoxicity in the endoplasmic reticulum: lessons from the Akita diabetic mouse. J Clin Invest. 2002;109(4):443–5. https://doi.org/10.1172/JCI15020.
38. Haseyama T, Fujita T, Hirasawa F, Tsukada M, Wakui H, Komatsuda A, et al. Complications of IgA nephropathy in a non-insulin-dependent diabetes model, the Akita mouse. Tohoku J Exp Med. 2002;198(4):233–44.
39. Alpers CE, Hudkins KL. Mouse models of diabetic nephropathy. Curr Opin Nephrol Hypertens. 2011;20(3):278–84. https://doi.org/10.1097/MNH.0b013e3283451901.
40. Gurley SB, Clare SE, Snow KP, Hu A, Meyer TW, Coffman TM. Impact of genetic background on nephropathy in diabetic mice. Am J Physiol Renal Physiol. 2006;290(1):F214–22. https://doi.org/10.1152/ajprenal.00204.2005.
41. Kakoki M, Kizer CM, Yi X, Takahashi N, Kim HS, Bagnell CR, et al. Senescence-associated phenotypes in Akita diabetic mice are enhanced by absence of bradykinin B2 receptors. J Clin Invest. 2006;116(5):1302–9. https://doi.org/10.1172/JCI26958.
42. Shi Y, Lo CS, Padda R, Abdo S, Chenier I, Filep JG, et al. Angiotensin-(1-7) prevents systemic hypertension, attenuates oxidative stress and tubulointerstitial fibrosis, and normalizes renal angiotensin-converting enzyme 2 and Mas receptor expression in diabetic mice. Clin Sci (Lond). 2015;128(10):649–63. https://doi.org/10.1042/CS20140329.
43. Liu GC, Fang F, Zhou J, Koulajian K, Yang S, Lam L, et al. Deletion of p47phox attenuates the progression of diabetic nephropathy and reduces the severity of diabetes in the Akita mouse. Diabetologia. 2012;55(9):2522–32. https://doi.org/10.1007/s00125-012-2586-1.

44. Fang F, Bae EH, Hu A, Liu GC, Zhou X, Williams V, et al. Deletion of the gene for adiponectin accelerates diabetic nephropathy in the Ins2 (+/C96Y) mouse. Diabetologia. 2015;58(7):1668–78. https://doi.org/10.1007/s00125-015-3605-9.
45. Fujita H, Fujishima H, Morii T, Sakamoto T, Komatsu K, Hosoba M, et al. Modulation of renal superoxide dismutase by telmisartan therapy in C57BL/6-Ins2(Akita) diabetic mice. Hypertens Res. 2012;35(2):213–20. https://doi.org/10.1038/hr.2011.176.
46. Proctor G, Jiang T, Iwahashi M, Wang Z, Li J, Levi M. Regulation of renal fatty acid and cholesterol metabolism, inflammation, and fibrosis in Akita and OVE26 mice with type 1 diabetes. Diabetes. 2006;55(9):2502–9. https://doi.org/10.2337/db05-0603.
47. Lee EY, Chung CH, Choi SO. Immunoglobulin A nephropathy in patients with non-insulin dependent diabetes mellitus. J Korean Med Sci. 1999;14(5):582–5. https://doi.org/10.3346/jkms.1999.14.5.582.
48. Zheng S, Noonan WT, Metreveli NS, Coventry S, Kralik PM, Carlson EC, et al. Development of late-stage diabetic nephropathy in OVE26 diabetic mice. Diabetes. 2004;53(12):3248–57.
49. Carlson EC, Audette JL, Klevay LM, Nguyen H, Epstein PN. Ultrastructural and functional analyses of nephropathy in calmodulin-induced diabetic transgenic mice. Anat Rec. 1997;247(1):9–19.
50. Carlson EC, Audette JL, Veitenheimer NJ, Risan JA, Laturnus DI, Epstein PN. Ultrastructural morphometry of capillary basement membrane thickness in normal and transgenic diabetic mice. Anat Rec A Discov Mol Cell Evol Biol. 2003;271(2):332–41. https://doi.org/10.1002/ar.a.10038.
51. Teiken JM, Audettey JL, Laturnus DI, Zheng S, Epstein PN, Carlson EC. Podocyte loss in aging OVE26 diabetic mice. Anat Rec (Hoboken). 2008;291(1):114–21. https://doi.org/10.1002/ar.20625.
52. Tsunekawa S, Miura Y, Yamamoto N, Itoh Y, Ariyoshi Y, Senda T, et al. Systemic administration of pituitary adenylate cyclase-activating polypeptide maintains beta-cell mass and retards onset of hyperglycaemia in beta-cell-specific calmodulin-overexpressing transgenic mice. Eur J Endocrinol. 2005;152(5):805–11. https://doi.org/10.1530/eje.1.01909.
53. Tsunekawa S, Yamamoto N, Tsukamoto K, Itoh Y, Kaneko Y, Kimura T, et al. Protection of pancreatic beta-cells by exendin-4 may involve the reduction of endoplasmic reticulum stress; in vivo and in vitro studies. J Endocrinol. 2007;193(1):65–74. https://doi.org/10.1677/JOE-06-0148.
54. Xu J, Huang Y, Li F, Zheng S, Epstein PN. FVB mouse genotype confers susceptibility to OVE26 diabetic albuminuria. Am J Physiol Renal Physiol. 2010;299(3):F487–94. https://doi.org/10.1152/ajprenal.00018.2010.
55. Epstein PN, Overbeek PA, Means AR. Calmodulin-induced early-onset diabetes in transgenic mice. Cell. 1989;58(6):1067–73.
56. Epstein PN, Ribar TJ, Decker GL, Yaney G, Means AR. Elevated beta-cell calmodulin produces a unique insulin secretory defect in transgenic mice. Endocrinology. 1992;130(3):1387–93. https://doi.org/10.1210/endo.130.3.1371447.
57. Yu W, Niwa T, Miura Y, Horio F, Teradaira S, Ribar TJ, et al. Calmodulin overexpression causes Ca(2+)-dependent apoptosis of pancreatic beta cells, which can be prevented by inhibition of nitric oxide synthase. Lab Invest. 2002;82(9):1229–39.
58. Yuzawa Y, Niki I, Kosugi T, Maruyama S, Yoshida F, Takeda M, et al. Overexpression of calmodulin in pancreatic beta cells induces diabetic nephropathy. J Am Soc Nephrol. 2008;19(9):1701–11. https://doi.org/10.1681/ASN.2006121358.
59. Zheng S, Carlson EC, Yang L, Kralik PM, Huang Y, Epstein PN. Podocyte-specific overexpression of the antioxidant metallothionein reduces diabetic nephropathy. J Am Soc Nephrol. 2008;19(11):2077–85. https://doi.org/10.1681/ASN.2007080967.
60. Breyer MD. Stacking the deck for drug discovery in diabetic nephropathy: in search of an animal model. J Am Soc Nephrol. 2008;19(9):1623–4. https://doi.org/10.1681/ASN.2008070705.

61. Hudkins KL, Pichaiwong W, Wietecha T, Kowalewska J, Banas MC, Spencer MW, et al. BTBR Ob/Ob mutant mice model progressive diabetic nephropathy. J Am Soc Nephrol. 2010;21(9):1533–42. https://doi.org/10.1681/ASN.2009121290.
62. Clee SM, Attie AD. The genetic landscape of type 2 diabetes in mice. Endocr Rev. 2007;28(1):48–83. https://doi.org/10.1210/er.2006-0035.
63. Clee SM, Nadler ST, Attie AD. Genetic and genomic studies of the BTBR ob/ob mouse model of type 2 diabetes. Am J Ther. 2005;12(6):491–8.
64. Betz B, Conway BR. Recent advances in animal models of diabetic nephropathy. Nephron Exp Nephrol. 2014;126(4):191–5. https://doi.org/10.1159/000363300.
65. Pichaiwong W, Hudkins KL, Wietecha T, Nguyen TQ, Tachaudomdach C, Li W, et al. Reversibility of structural and functional damage in a model of advanced diabetic nephropathy. J Am Soc Nephrol. 2013;24(7):1088–102. https://doi.org/10.1681/ASN.2012050445.
66. Tesch GH, Lim AK. Recent insights into diabetic renal injury from the db/db mouse model of type 2 diabetic nephropathy. Am J Physiol Renal Physiol. 2011;300(2):F301–10. https://doi.org/10.1152/ajprenal.00607.2010.
67. Chen H, Charlat O, Tartaglia LA, Woolf EA, Weng X, Ellis SJ, et al. Evidence that the diabetes gene encodes the leptin receptor: identification of a mutation in the leptin receptor gene in db/db mice. Cell. 1996;84(3):491–5.
68. Lee GH, Proenca R, Montez JM, Carroll KM, Darvishzadeh JG, Lee JI, et al. Abnormal splicing of the leptin receptor in diabetic mice. Nature. 1996;379(6566):632–5. https://doi.org/10.1038/379632a0.
69. Hummel KP, Dickie MM, Coleman DL. Diabetes, a new mutation in the mouse. Science. 1966;153(3740):1127–8.
70. Hummel KP, Coleman DL, Lane PW. The influence of genetic background on expression of mutations at the diabetes locus in the mouse. I. C57BL-KsJ and C57BL-6J strains. Biochem Genet. 1972;7(1):1–13.
71. Lee SM, Bressler R. Prevention of diabetic nephropathy by diet control in the db/db mouse. Diabetes. 1981;30(2):106–11.
72. Hong SW, Isono M, Chen S, Iglesias-De La Cruz MC, Han DC, Ziyadeh FN. Increased glomerular and tubular expression of transforming growth factor-beta1, its type II receptor, and activation of the Smad signaling pathway in the db/db mouse. Am J Pathol. 2001;158(5):1653–63.
73. Like AA, Lavine RL, Poffenbarger PL, Chick WL. Studies in the diabetic mutant mouse. VI. Evolution of glomerular lesions and associated proteinuria. Am J Pathol. 1972;66(2):193–224.
74. Lubec B, Rokitansky A, Hayde M, Aufricht C, Wagner U, Mallinger WR, et al. Thiaproline reduces glomerular basement membrane thickness and collagen accumulation in the db/db mouse. Nephron. 1994;66(3):333–6. https://doi.org/10.1159/000187832.
75. Koya D, Haneda M, Nakagawa H, Isshiki K, Sato H, Maeda S, et al. Amelioration of accelerated diabetic mesangial expansion by treatment with a PKC beta inhibitor in diabetic db/db mice, a rodent model for type 2 diabetes. FASEB J. 2000;14(3):439–47.
76. Kitada M, Kume S, Imaizumi N, Koya D. Resveratrol improves oxidative stress and protects against diabetic nephropathy through normalization of Mn-SOD dysfunction in AMPK/SIRT1-independent pathway. Diabetes. 2011;60(2):634–43. https://doi.org/10.2337/db10-0386.
77. Sharma K, McCue P, Dunn SR. Diabetic kidney disease in the db/db mouse. Am J Physiol Renal Physiol. 2003;284(6):F1138–44. https://doi.org/10.1152/ajprenal.00315.2002.
78. Mauer SM, Steffes MW, Brown DM. The kidney in diabetes. Am J Med. 1981;70(3):603–12.
79. Mauer SM, Steffes MW, Ellis EN, Sutherland DE, Brown DM, Goetz FC. Structural-functional relationships in diabetic nephropathy. J Clin Invest. 1984;74(4):1143–55. https://doi.org/10.1172/JCI111523.
80. Osterby R. A quantitative electron microscopic study of mesangial regions in glomeruli from patients with short term juvenile diabetes mellitus. Lab Invest. 1973;29(1):99–110.

81. Steffes MW, Osterby R, Chavers B, Mauer SM. Mesangial expansion as a central mechanism for loss of kidney function in diabetic patients. Diabetes. 1989;38(9):1077–81.
82. Cohen MP, Sharma K, Jin Y, Hud E, Wu VY, Tomaszewski J, et al. Prevention of diabetic nephropathy in db/db mice with glycated albumin antagonists. A novel treatment strategy. J Clin Invest. 1995;95(5):2338–45. https://doi.org/10.1172/JCI117926.
83. Ha TS, Barnes JL, Stewart JL, Ko CW, Miner JH, Abrahamson DR, et al. Regulation of renal laminin in mice with type II diabetes. J Am Soc Nephrol. 1999;10(9):1931–9.
84. Riser BL, Denichilo M, Cortes P, Baker C, Grondin JM, Yee J, et al. Regulation of connective tissue growth factor activity in cultured rat mesangial cells and its expression in experimental diabetic glomerulosclerosis. J Am Soc Nephrol. 2000;11(1):25–38.
85. Ziyadeh FN, Hoffman BB, Han DC, Iglesias-De La Cruz MC, Hong SW, Isono M, et al. Long-term prevention of renal insufficiency, excess matrix gene expression, and glomerular mesangial matrix expansion by treatment with monoclonal antitransforming growth factor-beta antibody in db/db diabetic mice. Proc Natl Acad Sci USA. 2000;97(14):8015–20. https://doi.org/10.1073/pnas.120055097.
86. Mohan S, Reddick RL, Musi N, Horn DA, Yan B, Prihoda TJ, et al. Diabetic eNOS knockout mice develop distinct macro- and microvascular complications. Lab Invest. 2008;88(5):515–28. https://doi.org/10.1038/labinvest.2008.23.
87. Zhao HJ, Wang S, Cheng H, Zhang MZ, Takahashi T, Fogo AB, et al. Endothelial nitric oxide synthase deficiency produces accelerated nephropathy in diabetic mice. J Am Soc Nephrol. 2006;17(10):2664–9. https://doi.org/10.1681/ASN.2006070798.
88. Watanabe Y, Hotta N. [Tubulointerstitial injury in diabetes mellitus (including Armanni-Ebstein lesion)]. Ryoikibetsu Shokogun Shirizu.1997;(17 Pt 2):225–8.
89. Tomino Y. Lessons from the KK-Ay mouse, a spontaneous animal model for the treatment of human type 2 diabetic nephropathy. Nephrourol Mon. 2012;4(3):524–9. https://doi.org/10.5812/numonthly.1954.
90. Omote K, Gohda T, Murakoshi M, Sasaki Y, Kazuno S, Fujimura T, et al. Role of the TNF pathway in the progression of diabetic nephropathy in KK-A(y) mice. Am J Physiol Renal Physiol. 2014;306(11):F1335–47. https://doi.org/10.1152/ajprenal.00509.2013.
91. Ito T, Tanimoto M, Yamada K, Kaneko S, Matsumoto M, Obayashi K, et al. Glomerular changes in the KK-Ay/Ta mouse: a possible model for human type 2 diabetic nephropathy. Nephrology (Carlton). 2006;11(1):29–35. https://doi.org/10.1111/j.1440-1797.2006.00543.x.
92. Matsumoto M, Tanimoto M, Gohda T, Aoki T, Murakoshi M, Yamada K, et al. Effect of pitavastatin on type 2 diabetes mellitus nephropathy in KK-Ay/Ta mice. Metab Clin Exp. 2008;57(5):691–7. https://doi.org/10.1016/j.metabol.2008.01.007.
93. Heinonen SE, Genove G, Bengtsson E, Hubschle T, Akesson L, Hiss K, et al. Animal models of diabetic macrovascular complications: key players in the development of new therapeutic approaches. J Diabetes Res. 2015;2015:404085. https://doi.org/10.1155/2015/404085.
94. Shiota M, Printz RL. Diabetes in Zucker diabetic fatty rat. Methods Mol Biol. 2012;933:103–23. https://doi.org/10.1007/978-1-62703-068-7_8.
95. Phillips MS, Liu Q, Hammond HA, Dugan V, Hey PJ, Caskey CJ, et al. Leptin receptor missense mutation in the fatty Zucker rat. Nat Genet. 1996;13(1):18–9. https://doi.org/10.1038/ng0596-18.
96. Katsuda Y, Ohta T, Miyajima K, Kemmochi Y, Sasase T, Tong B, et al. Diabetic complications in obese type 2 diabetic rat models. Exp Anim. 2014;63(2):121–32.
97. Vora JP, Zimsen SM, Houghton DC, Anderson S. Evolution of metabolic and renal changes in the ZDF/Drt-fa rat model of type II diabetes. J Am Soc Nephrol. 1996;7(1):113–7.
98. Takiyama Y, Harumi T, Watanabe J, Fujita Y, Honjo J, Shimizu N, et al. Tubular injury in a rat model of type 2 diabetes is prevented by metformin: a possible role of HIF-1alpha expression and oxygen metabolism. Diabetes. 2011;60(3):981–92. https://doi.org/10.2337/db10-0655.
99. Kawano K, Hirashima T, Mori S, Saitoh Y, Kurosumi M, Natori T. Spontaneous long-term hyperglycemic rat with diabetic complications. Otsuka Long-Evans Tokushima Fatty (OLETF) strain. Diabetes. 1992;41(11):1422–8.

100. Nagai N, Ito Y. Therapeutic effects of sericin on diabetic keratopathy in Otsuka Long-Evans Tokushima Fatty rats. World J Diabetes. 2013;4(6):282–9. https://doi.org/10.4239/wjd.v4.i6.282.
101. Nagai N, Murao T, Ito Y, Okamoto N, Sasaki M. Enhancing effects of sericin on corneal wound healing in Otsuka Long-Evans Tokushima fatty rats as a model of human type 2 diabetes. Biol Pharm Bull. 2009;32(9):1594–9.
102. Lee EY, Kim GT, Hyun M, Kim S, Seok S, Choi R, et al. Peroxisome proliferator-activated receptor-delta activation ameliorates albuminuria by preventing nephrin loss and restoring podocyte integrity in type 2 diabetes. Nephrol Dial Transplant. 2012;27(11):4069–79. https://doi.org/10.1093/ndt/gfs358.
103. Goto Y, Kakizaki M, Masaki N. Production of spontaneous diabetic rats by repetition of selective breeding. Tohoku J Exp Med. 1976;119(1):85–90.
104. Ostenson CG, Khan A, Abdel-Halim SM, Guenifi A, Suzuki K, Goto Y, et al. Abnormal insulin secretion and glucose metabolism in pancreatic islets from the spontaneously diabetic GK rat. Diabetologia. 1993;36(1):3–8.
105. Yagihashi S, Goto Y, Kakizaki M, Kaseda N. Thickening of glomerular basement membrane in spontaneously diabetic rats. Diabetologia. 1978;15(4):309–12.
106. Feng B, Yan XF, Xue JL, Xu L, Wang H. The protective effects of alpha-lipoic acid on kidneys in type 2 diabetic Goto-Kakisaki rats via reducing oxidative stress. Int J Mol Sci. 2013;14(4):6746–56. https://doi.org/10.3390/ijms14046746.
107. Chen S, Yang T, Liu F, Li H, Guo Y, Yang H, et al. Inflammatory factor-specific sumoylation regulates NF-kappaB signalling in glomerular cells from diabetic rats. Inflamm Res. 2014;63(1):23–31. https://doi.org/10.1007/s00011-013-0675-3.
108. Wang Y, Nie M, Lu Y, Wang R, Li J, Yang B, et al. Fucoidan exerts protective effects against diabetic nephropathy related to spontaneous diabetes through the NF-kappaB signaling pathway in vivo and in vitro. Int J Mol Med. 2015;35(4):1067–73. https://doi.org/10.3892/ijmm.2015.2095.
109. Kojima N, Slaughter TN, Paige A, Kato S, Roman RJ, Williams JM. Comparison of the development diabetic induced renal disease in strains of Goto-Kakizaki rats. J Diabetes Metab. 2013;Suppl 9(5):S9-005. https://doi.org/10.4172/2155-6156.S9-005.
110. Akimoto T, Nakama K, Katsuta Y, Zhang XJ, Ohsuga M, Ishizaki M, et al. Characterization of a novel congenic strain of diabetic fatty (WBN/Kob-Lepr(fa)) rat. Biochem Biophys Res Commun. 2008;366(2):556–62. https://doi.org/10.1016/j.bbrc.2007.12.003.
111. Ohashi K, Kim JH, Hara H, Aso R, Akimoto T, Nakama K. WBN/Kob rats. A new spontaneously occurring model of chronic pancreatitis. Int J Pancreatol. 1990;6(4):231–47.
112. Takagi Y, Kadowaki H, Kobayashi I, Ito K, Ito K, Shirai M, et al. Effects of high-sodium intake on systemic blood pressure and vascular responses in spontaneously diabetic WBN/Kob-Lepr(fa/fa) rats. Clin Exp Pharmacol Physiol. 2017;44(2):305–12. https://doi.org/10.1111/1440-1681.12700.

MIX
Papier aus verantwortungsvollen Quellen
Paper from responsible sources
FSC® C105338

If you have any concerns about our products,
you can contact us on
ProductSafety@springernature.com

In case Publisher is established outside the EU,
the EU authorized representative is:
Springer Nature Customer Service Center GmbH
Europaplatz 3, 69115 Heidelberg, Germany

Printed by Libri Plureos GmbH
in Hamburg, Germany